A PARENT'S GUIDE TO

RHEUMATIC DISEASES
IN CHILDREN

A PARENT'S GUIDE TO

RHEUMATIC DISEASES IN CHILDREN

Thomas J. A. Lehman, M.D., F.A.A.P., F.A.C.R.

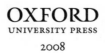

OXFORD
UNIVERSITY PRESS
2008

OXFORD
UNIVERSITY PRESS

Oxford University Press, Inc., publishes works that further
Oxford University's objective of excellence
in research, scholarship, and education.

Oxford New York
Auckland   Cape Town   Dar es Salaam   Hong Kong   Karachi
Kuala Lumpur   Madrid   Melbourne   Mexico City   Nairobi
New Delhi   Shanghai   Taipei   Toronto

With offices in
Argentina   Austria   Brazil   Chile   Czech Republic   France   Greece
Guatemala   Hungary   Italy   Japan   Poland   Portugal   Singapore
South Korea   Switzerland   Thailand   Turkey   Ukraine   Vietnam

Published by Oxford University Press, Inc.
198 Madison Avenue, New York, New York 10016
www.oup.com

Oxford is a registered trademark of Oxford University Press

Library of Congress Cataloging-in-Publication Data
Lehman, Thomas J.A.
A parent's guide to rheumatic diseases in children/ Thomas J.A.
Lehman.
p. cm.
Includes index.
ISBN 978-0-19-534189-8 (pbk.)
1.   Pediatric rheumatology–Popular works.
2.   Rheumatism in children–Popular works.
I.   Title.
RJ482.R48L449 2008
618.92'723—dc22
2007046611

9 8 7 6 5 4 3 2 1
Printed in the United States of America
on acid-free paper

Dedication

This book is dedicated to the many children around the world who have muscle, bone, or joint pain, or who have arthritis—and to their families and those who care for them. It will help you understand whether your child is being properly diagnosed and cared for and the importance of proper care. This book is derived from *It's Not Just Growing Pains*, but it has been rewritten to improve its usefulness to parents and highlight the most recent information on diagnosis and treatment. This is not a book just for parents who know their children have arthritis or a related condition. This is also a book for parents of children with complaints, discomfort, or disability who are not getting the answers they need from their physicians.

This book is dedicated as well to those physicians who inspired me to become a physician and scientist with the goal of providing the best possible care to children with complicated and often chronic conditions: Dr. Harry O. Zamkin, a pediatrician who loved his patients; Dr. Virgil Hanson, a pediatric rheumatologist who taught that pediatric rheumatology is not learned from textbooks—it is learned by listening and carefully evaluating the children you treat, every time you see them; Dr. Barbara Ansell, a pediatric rheumatologist who taught that an "atypical case of A" was most likely a "typical case of B" that I had not thought of, and so much more; Dr. Arthur D. Schwabe, a gastroenterologist who taught me to never stop asking questions of the children, their families, and myself until all the answers fit together and made sense; Dr. John Decker, for many years the "dean" of rheumatology at the National Institutes of Health in Bethesda, Maryland, who inspired so many by his quiet confidence combined with a willingness to endorse any idea that seemed sensible, no matter that it had never been done before; and Dr. Jack Klippel, for continuing to say, "If not you, who? It's your idea—do it." In the 1960s and 1970s, when these physicians were in active practice, the emphasis was on making the situation better. Now, in the early 2000s, we are beginning to consider the possibility of cures.

Contents

PART III: LIVING WITH A CHILD WHO HAS A CHRONIC CONDITION

Introduction

I am writing this book in the hope that it will speed the proper diagnosis and treatment of children with rheumatic disease. The pages that follow are based on my thirty years of experience and will provide the information you need to understand what is happening to your child and your family, and what you need to do to get the best outcome.

One of the questions parents most frequently ask me as they come to grips with their child's diagnosis of rheumatic disease is "Why did this happen?" Medical research has made great strides over the past fifty years, but we still can't really answer this question. From the immune system's point of view, there are all sorts of bad guys out there—bacteria, viruses, parasites, and so on. The immune system's job is to provide us with a strong defense against these threats, but sometimes its response is *too* strong. It overreacts to normal tissue as if there were disease, causing unintended damage in the process. Rheumatic diseases appear to be the result of this immune overreaction. Why exactly this occurs in some people and not in others is still unknown. We do know, however, that there is probably some genetic component, since most of the rheumatic diseases clearly occur with increased frequency in relatives of people with the diseases.

In this day and age, millions of dollars are spent annually on research into causes of diseases such as these, as well as potential treatments. Still, the most common cause of a child doing poorly today is that too much time elapsed before he or she received proper medical attention. Parents must make sure their children are seen by experienced physicians familiar with childhood arthritis and related diseases, but parents must also ensure that their children do the exercises, take the medicines, get the blood tests, and keep their appointments. The key to getting the best possible outcome for children with rheumatic disease is for parents and physicians to work together to do whatever is necessary. If you realize that you cannot work well with your physician, find another.

Much of the information in this book is not available in today's textbooks, and in many cases the treatments recommended have not yet been subjected to rigorous clinical trials. That does not mean that what you read here is incorrect, useless, or harmful. It is important to understand that large-scale controlled trials require huge numbers of study participants, and there are far too few children with rheumatic disease for researchers to study any but the most basic questions. Furthermore, such rigorous studies take five to ten years to carry out, and your child can't wait that long to start treatment. Given these facts, what parents and children need most today is the advice of an experienced specialist in the field who has seen which treatments give the best long-term results.

The care of children with muscle, bone, and joint pain is still more an art than a science. Obtaining the best possible results depends far more on experience, careful monitoring, and minor adjustments than on strict adherence to a standard protocol. Certainly not every physician will share my opinions, and not every physician is willing to go beyond the proven in reaching for the best possible outcome. But the final decisions will always be yours.

How to Use This Book

If you are the parent of a child who has been given a diagnosis, you should begin by reading about that diagnosis to see whether it accurately describes your child's symptoms. For parents who know their child's diagnosis, this book has useful chapters on the latest medications, the meaning of laboratory test results, family issues, getting the best care for your child, and reconstructive surgery. You will find a lot of information that will allow you to make informed choices.

If you are the parent of a child who does not have a diagnosis, or the diagnosis you have been given does not seem correct to you, you should begin with Chapter 2, "Figuring Out What's Wrong." It is my goal to help you think about what the correct answer might be. Then you should approach your physician and discuss your thoughts. Most physicians will be happy to discuss the situation with you, to help you to understand why the diagnosis is correct or to rethink the diagnosis with you.

This book will help you to understand why physicians ask the questions they ask, and perhaps what questions they should have asked but didn't. Don't be afraid to volunteer information that the physician didn't ask for. Many physicians' offices have taken to using forms you fill out before you see the doctor. Make sure you think for a minute before answering the questions, and ask the doctor about any question you are unsure of. I prefer not to use those forms because in discussion with parents I often learn details that the parents thought were unimportant and would not have indicated on a form. Make sure your child is getting the time and attention needed. If you are still dissatisfied after discussing your child's care with your physician, see Chapter 25, "Getting the Best Results for Your Child."

PART I

MY CHILD
COMPLAINS OF PAIN

1

Growing Pains?

Whenever a child limps or complains that an arm or leg hurts, our first thought is that he or she must have injured it, even if the child does not remember having done so. The family is likely to seek medical advice only if the pain is very severe or persists for more than a day or two. Even when the pain or limp continues beyond a few days, many parents and physicians dismiss the problem as growing pains. Children do have growing pains; in fact, they are fairly common. Unfortunately, many children with serious problems are misdiagnosed with growing pains for weeks or even months.

Growing pains typically occur in young children between the ages of three and eight years. The child will wake up suddenly, complaining that his or her legs hurt. Most often the episode occurs during the first few hours after the child has gone to sleep, but it can occur in the middle of the night. Typically, when asked where it hurts, the child will point to the front or back of the knee, or the muscles just above the knee. The pain will usually disappear with ten or fifteen minutes of gentle massage and be completely gone in the morning. The pain is almost always in a large joint such as the knee, not a finger or toe. Sometimes the pains will wake the child up two or three nights in a row, but more often they occur episodically over a period of weeks or months. Growing pains occur most often during periods of rapid growth and after days of extra physical activity (when they may be joined by muscle complaints). They may disappear for months or a year only to start up again during another period of rapid growth.

The key is that the child is absolutely fine when he or she wakes up in the morning. There is no pain, limp, or any other abnormality. If the child has any pain when he or she wakes up in the morning or during the day, this should not be dismissed as growing pains. Minor pains are common and most often not due to a serious condition, but they are not growing pains.

Doctors are not in complete agreement regarding the cause of growing pains. There is evidence that the body produces more growth hormone at night, and some doctors believe the body is actually growing faster at night, leading to the pain. A more likely explanation is related to the gate control theory of pain.

While the brain is constantly receiving sensory input from all parts of the body at all times, the center in the brain that receives this information filters it and decides what to bring to your conscious attention and what you can ignore. During the day, when children are awake and active, any message to the brain about pain from tendons and muscles being stretched by growth is lost among the sensory input from all the other things that are going on—watching, listening, touching, exploring, moving around. But when a child is falling asleep at night and there are no distractions, the pain impulses from the muscles and tendons may be passed on to the higher brain centers, causing the child to wake up.

Surprisingly, growing pains tend to run in families. If one of your children is having a lot of growing pains, ask your parents and your spouse's parents. It's likely one of you also had a lot of growing pains.

For a child with typical growing pains, a trip to the doctor is not usually necessary. A child who has typical nighttime pain and is always fine in the morning can usually be treated with gentle reassurance, massage, or, if the pain is more severe, a dose of acetaminophen or ibuprofen. If a child wakes up with pain several nights in a row, it may be helpful to give a dose of medication at bedtime to decrease the perception of pain and prevent the child from waking up; after two or three nights without episodes, the medication should be stopped. However, if the pains persist despite medication or return as soon as the medication is stopped, a full medical evaluation should be done.

Children with growing pains should have absolutely normal blood tests and X-rays. Bone scans, magnetic resonance imaging (MRI), and other special tests are not necessary for a child with growing pains. But they may be necessary to exclude other causes of pain in children who have atypical findings, persistent pain, or pain during the day.

Growing pains will go away. They may come back when the child goes through another period of rapid growth, but they never stay. While inconvenient, they are not of any long-term significance. They do not interfere with proper growth or development. And remember, growing pains never occur during the day. Any child who complains of pain during the day should be seen by a physician.

2

Figuring Out What's Wrong

When a child has muscle, bone, or joint pain, it is important to understand that each of the conditions that may be responsible has a typical set of problems it causes (symptoms), a typical age group in which it occurs, and other typical findings that usually make it easy for an experienced physician to diagnose. At the same time, if a child does not have the typical problems or is not the typical age, it's much less likely that the suspected condition is the proper explanation. This is why your physician should always start the evaluation by asking you (and your child, if he or she is old enough) questions about the problem.

GIVING YOUR CHILD'S HISTORY

As a parent evaluating your own child, ask yourself these questions and think about the answers. Your physician will want to know the answers to help arrive at an appropriate diagnosis. In addition, knowing the answers to these questions and what diseases they suggest will help you decide whether the physician's diagnosis makes sense to you. If it does not, discuss what you have noticed with your physician. If the physician is not interested in your child's history, something's wrong.

The first thing you should have in mind when you go to the doctor's office is your chief complaint. What is it that you want the doctor to fix? Do not tell the doctor things other doctors have told you. Tell the doctor what the problem is as clearly as you can, for example, "My daughter's left knee hurts." Sometimes the problem is more general: "My son aches all over and feels very weak." If your child is old enough to explain, let him or her answer the questions in the doctor's office. You may have to help out, but often children can provide the doctor with meaningful information the parents weren't aware of. For teenagers in particular, it is very important to let them explain their own problems. You may have to help out, but let them go first.

The key pieces of information for the physician often can be summarized in just a few words.

- *Quality of the pain.* What does the pain feel like? Is it a sharp pain or a dull ache?
- *Location of the pain.* Some problems cause the front of the knee to hurt; others cause pain in the side of the knee. Sometimes the pain is above the knee; sometimes it's below. Each suggests a different diagnosis.
- *Duration of the pain.* How long has the pain been going on, and how did it start?
- *Whether the pain is changing.* Is it getting better over time or worse?
- *What lessens the pain and what makes it worse?* Is it the same all day long, or does it vary with activities?

These sound like simple questions, but for an experienced physician they can rapidly lead to the diagnosis. Imagine a fourteen-year-old boy is brought to the doctor because his knee hurts. If the boy says, "My knee hurts all the time," the doctor doesn't have much information to go on. "It hurts when I walk on it" does not tell us very much, either. But if the boy says, "Most of the time I'm fine, but when I put my foot down and turn to the left, I get a sudden sharp pain on the side of my knee. After five or ten minutes the pain gets better, but then it happens again if I put my foot down and turn left again," this clearly suggests a mechanical problem in the knee, probably a torn meniscus.

With knee problems, for example, the doctor needs to know if the knee is stiff when the child wakes up in the morning or whether it hurts only with activity. Sometimes the child and parents are not sure. An experienced physician will ask the same question several different ways: "Are you stiff when you wake up in the morning? Do you have trouble getting out of the car after a long car ride? Do you have trouble getting out of your seat in the movie theater after a long movie? Suppose you and I are walking in a shopping center—how far can you walk without stopping? If we stop and sit, does your knee immediately get better or does it take five or ten minutes to get better? If we get up to go again after your knee has improved, does it start to hurt immediately and get worse? Does it seem stiff, but then get better after a few steps? Is it fine until we've been walking for ten or fifteen minutes again?" The answers to these questions will help the physician determine the correct diagnosis.

Mechanical problems often cause pain after a period of use. They get better with rest. Then they start to hurt again after another period of use. Arthritis may begin to hurt after a period of use and then get better with rest as well; however, children with arthritis will be stiff when they get up to walk again but improve after a few steps. The child with arthritis will often describe trouble with long car rides or sitting in a movie theater, while children with injuries are much less likely to do so.

Sometimes the questioning needs to go in a different direction. A child with chondromalacia patella (a mechanical irritation of the knee; see Chapter 3) may be brought to the physician's office with the same chief complaint, knee pain. There is no suggestion of stiffness, but it hurts when she walks long distances. If you ask whether it hurts more going up- or downstairs, children with chondromalacia patella characteristically complain of more pain going downstairs. In contrast, children with unrecognized dermatomyositis (see Chapter 14) might also complain of leg or knee pain, but they will have much more trouble going upstairs. Knowing that one child has more trouble going upstairs and the other more trouble going downstairs helps to guide the evaluation and eliminate unnecessary tests.

Another important question is how the pain began. If the child says, "My knee hurt immediately after I was tackled during a football game," the list of possible causes is very different than for the child who cannot explain how the pain began. At the same time, you need to be very careful about injury as the explanation. I have seen parents bring in small children and even teenagers with a swollen finger or toe and say, "We did not see anything, but we assumed she must have jammed it." Typically, children who have injured a finger or toe badly enough for it to be significantly swollen know exactly what happened. But children with arthritis or other diseases cannot tell you exactly how or when it started; they (or their parents) just assume they must have twisted it or otherwise somehow injured the joint. Children who exhibit an unexplained "sausage digit" often have psoriatic arthritis (see Chapter 7). I see many children with spondyloarthropathy who complain of repeatedly spraining their ankles or wrists but cannot really say when the injury occurred; it just happens "all the time." These are not sprains or fractures at all. Spondyloarthropathy is a type of arthritis that commonly causes tendons to be inflamed where they insert into the bone, mimicking a sprain or minor fracture.

Injuries

Most children with a definite history of injury have an orthopedic problem. These problems are usually easily diagnosed with some combination of history, physical examination, X-rays, ultrasound, or MRIs.

However, sometimes there is a definite history of injury that leads everyone in the wrong direction. A child may be brought to the emergency room limping because he or she fell a few days earlier and is not getting better. The X-ray evaluation may show arthritis or a bone infection, not an injury. We used to think that the child probably fell because of the infection or arthritis and that the fall brought attention to the problem. However, we now know that an initial injury can alter the dynamics of the bone and joint, making the child more vulnerable to infection or arthritis.

When I'm evaluating a child with pain that started on a certain day, I frequently ask about what happened in the days or weeks just before that. Infection-associated arthritis (Chapter 7) often begins ten to fourteen days after an episode of sore throat or flu. Another situation in which the history is important is making a diagnosis of plant thorn synovitis (Chapter 3). This type of arthritis occurs when a child falls on a palm frond, cactus thorn, or other sharp-edged warm-climate plant and a piece of the plant penetrates the knee and breaks off, remaining inside the knee. The fall usually took place six or eight weeks before the child developed symptoms. The family has no reason to think their trip to Florida in February has anything to do with the child's knee pain in April. As a result, they will not think to mention it unless asked about travel. There are many similar situations. You cannot always rely on the physician to remember to ask you about travel, unusual pets, or other findings that might be important. Tell the physician anything you think might be important.

Physicians do not know all about the lives of the children they are taking care of, and parents do not know what is important to the physician and what is not. The key to the best possible care is an open exchange of information. Often at the very end of a long history, a parent will say, "I don't know if this is important, but …" Surprisingly often, that may be the key piece of information that leads to an accurate diagnosis. To get this information, physicians will ask a lot of questions that may seem unrelated and unimportant: "Is the child growing well? Has there been any fever or rash? Has the child had frequent infections?" I ask all families these questions because I have no way of knowing in advance when the answers will make a difference. For example, children with chronic problems or severe problems often have been losing weight. Fevers or night sweats often suggest a long-standing problem, perhaps a more severe one. And children with a history of frequent ear or upper respiratory infections may have immunoglobulin A (IgA) deficiency or other immune deficiencies that are associated with an increased frequency of arthritis and other rheumatic diseases (see Chapter 7). All these questions may seem like a waste of time when your child's knee hurts and your answer is no, but they are very important when the answer is yes.

Medications

It is important to tell the physician about all the medications your child is taking, including vitamins, supplements, and any medications you obtained without a prescription. ("I gave Johnny one of Grandma's pills that she had left over from when she had bronchitis" can turn out to be the explanation for the entire problem if it's an allergic reaction to Grandma's medicine.) The physician needs to know what has been done to treat the problem in the past. He or she also needs to know what other medical problems the child is being treated for and how. Furthermore, the physician needs to be sure the child is not on a medication that may be causing the problem, including one that has recently been stopped. In addition, it is important for the physician to be sure that the child is not taking a medication that will interact with the medications the physician wants to prescribe. If your child is allergic to particular drugs, know which ones they are, and tell your doctor during the appointment. Let the physician know if other medications are added or changed while you are under his or her care. I've had problems where parents thought the medication I prescribed was causing a side effect, only to realize another doctor had recently added a medication that was well known for causing that side effect. Other times parents start children on medicines that shouldn't be used with the drugs I'm prescribing because they forgot to tell the regular doctor about the medications I've prescribed.

Past Medical History

This is another long set of questions that doctors ask and families frequently wonder about. The physician needs to know whether the child has other illnesses or conditions that may be related to the symptoms or relevant to the treatment. You should try to give the doctor as much information as possible. A child might be ten or eleven years old, but the strange problem he or she is having may be the result of something that happened in the neonatal intensive care unit shortly after birth. The physician cannot even begin to suspect that if he or she does not know that the child was in the neonatal intensive care unit. If your physician forgets to ask, it's a good idea to bring it up yourself.

Not long ago a child was sent to me because of blood in the urine and joint pains. The referring physician was worried about lupus. After I'd gotten all the relevant information from the mother and was asking about past medical problems, she told me the child had frequently been treated for an infected parotid gland. Then I asked the child whether he had trouble making tears or eating certain foods. As a result, I knew to evaluate him for Sjögren's syndrome. Despite several years of the child's being treated for various symptoms, the correct diagnosis had not been previously considered because no one obtained the pieces of information necessary to see how everything fit together to suggest this diagnosis.

Family History

This is one of the most important parts of evaluating children with chronic disease. Many diseases have a tendency to run in families. Often I request extra tests for a disease that I would not initially have suspected because there is a strong family history of the disease. I have discovered children with inflammatory bowel disease long before they were having abdominal symptoms because I requested the appropriate tests when I realized that they had joint pains and a family history of bowel disease. Celiac disease (in which the child cannot tolerate the gluten found in many grains), rheumatic fever, psoriatic arthritis, spondyloarthropathies, and many other diseases tend to run in families.

Social History

Many people think social history consists simply of asking where a child goes to school, what grade the child is in, and what the child wants to be when he or she grows up. But it also includes asking about smoking or alcohol and other drug use in teenagers. It means that I know whether a child lives at home or in a boarding school. Does the child come home to a parent or a babysitter or go to an after-school club? All these pieces of information may provide the answer to the problem. It's easy to consider psittacosis (pigeon fancier's disease) if you know that a child raises birds as a hobby or helps someone who does. But you have to ask about hobbies to know the answer.

Review of Systems

The review of systems is your doctor's last try to find out anything you forgot to mention. Is the child allergic to any drugs? Does the child have any bleeding problems? Are there any problems with the hair, eyes, or ears? I ask about everything from the top of the head to the bottom of the feet. No one—not the physician, the child, or the family—knows for sure whether the answer to the problem is going to become obvious from these questions. Often it does not, but we never know until we ask.

THE COMPLETE PHYSICAL EXAMINATION

If you have a child with an obvious injury to an arm or leg, then you want the physician to examine the limb carefully. However, if your child is having recurrent problems with injuries or has complaints without an obvious explanation, you want to be sure the child is examined completely. Physicians who are used to dealing with injuries often forget this.

There's no space in this book to go into the many specific findings that an experienced physician will look for during a physical examination, but as a parent, you can know whether the doctor evaluated your child completely or just looked at what hurts. Diagnosing illness is like solving puzzles—you'll never do a good job if you do not collect all the clues.

When your child is examined because of pain in the muscles, bone, or joints, there are several important steps in the evaluation.

- Is the pain in the joint (where the bones come together)?
- Is the pain just above or below the joint?
- Is their pain in the middle of the arm or leg—far away from a joint?
- Is the child in pain without being touched, or does the area hurt only if squeezed?
- Is this the only joint that hurts or do other joints hurt if squeezed?
- Is the area that hurts hot or warm to the touch?
- Is it red? Is it obviously swollen?
- Does the child have other findings (a rash, bumps, etc.)?
- Can the child bend the joint without pain and display the normal range of motion? (Healthy children are far more flexible than adults.)

As a parent, you are not expected to be able to do a careful examination yourself, but you should notice whether the physician did a careful examination of your child. If your child's problems aren't getting better, you want to be sure he or she has been properly evaluated.

LABORATORY TESTS AND OTHER EVALUATIONS

Proper diagnostic testing may include blood tests, X-rays (radiographs), bone scans, MRI, ultrasound (sonograms), and even biopsies of affected joints and tissues. Chapter 22 offers an extensive discussion of common laboratory and diagnostic tests. It is important to remember that diagnostic tests are not a substitute for knowledge and judgment. I often see children who previously have had thousands of dollars' worth of unnecessary tests, resulting in the wrong diagnosis. The key to proper diagnosis and treatment is a careful history and a thorough physical examination, as discussed above. After those have been done, appropriate diagnostic tests can help to pinpoint the cause of the problem and aid in planning treatment. Simply performing a large battery of poorly thought-out tests not only wastes time and money but also exposes the patient to unwarranted risks associated with both the testing procedures and the pursuit of false leads.

Proper evaluation consists of taking a careful history and doing a complete physical exam. In the hands of an experienced physician, this is often sufficient to establish the diagnosis. Further testing should be ordered only to confirm the diagnosis and ensure that there is nothing else wrong. Only if physicians are having difficulty finding the cause of a child's problems is a much more extensive evaluation warranted (see Chapter 4).

Even when appropriate tests are done, it is important to be sure they are properly interpreted. A ten-year-old boy was sent to me because of hip pain. The family brought an X-ray of the hip that had been interpreted by the radiologist as showing no hip damage. A bone scan of the hip was also done that showed no abnormal uptake in the hip, that is, no damage. When I examined the child, it was clear that his pain was not in the hip but adjacent to it. The X-ray and the bone scan brought to me by the family were indeed negative for hip damage, but both showed a fracture of the pubic ramus (a bone near the hip). Looking at just the hip, the doctors had overlooked the fracture nearby. The child pointed right to the location of the fracture when he was asked where it hurt.

3

Common Causes of Pain

KNEE PAIN

When evaluating a child with knee pain, it is important to separate mechanical problems from problems resulting from infections or inflammation. Know the answers to the following questions before you go to the doctor's office.

- Did the pain begin immediately after an injury? Or did your child begin complaining of pain without there having been an obvious injury?
- Does the knee hurt all the time?
- Does it hurt only in the middle of the night?
- Does it hurt only when the child is running (for example, during sports)?
- Does it hurt only in the evening?
- Can the child play for a time but then have to come off the field? If the child comes off the field, is he or she better in five minutes and back in the game, or is the child out for the rest of the day?
- When the child wakes up the next morning, does he or she feel better or worse?
- Is the knee stiff the next morning? Does it loosen up after the child gets up and gets going?
- Has the knee ever been swollen?
- Are any other joints ever stiff or swollen?
- Has there been any fever?
- Has there been any recent diarrhea or viral illness?

The answers to these questions will suggest a variety of different explanations for the pain. Knowing the answers in advance should help your doctor to pinpoint the problem quickly.

Children with mechanical problems typically hurt with activity. Stop the activity and the pain goes away; resume the activity and the pain comes back. If there is a fracture or an infection, the pain is there all the time. If there is a torn

13

ligament or meniscus, the pain may be intermittent. It will come on with activities and clear more slowly. Pain that begins with activity but does not disappear when the activity is stopped and often results in stiffness the next morning suggests arthritis, as does pain that comes and goes with changes in barometric pressure.

Sometimes a child's pain is thought to be the result of a fracture that is not visible on X-ray. It is true that some fractures may be very small and not evident in a first X-ray. However, as the bone heals, it will form a large callus that will easily be seen on a follow-up X-ray. Other children with pain are thought to have a growth plate injury that is hard to see on the X-ray. The growth plate is the junction between the shaft and the end of the bone where rapid growth is occurring. If a fracture is seen or suspected, the child will be put in a cast for an appropriate period. Following cast removal, the child should recover quickly. Repeated injuries in which the fractures are hard to see should be regarded with suspicion. Many children with arthritis are originally incorrectly diagnosed with "small fractures."

If the X-rays are negative, the child may be diagnosed with a sprain (a partial tear of the ligament holding two bones in proper alignment). Often the symptoms will go away quickly with use of an elastic bandage and crutches or a walking boot. However, injuries to the supporting ligaments of the knee or to a meniscus (the button-shaped cartilage shock absorber found on top of the tibia that absorb the downward pressure from the femur) will require further attention. And any child with recurrent injuries of this type needs careful medical evaluation to determine why they keep occurring.

If a child continues to have knee pain after the initial treatment, a thorough repeat evaluation should be done. It is also important for the physician to determine whether it is in fact the knee joint that is the source of the pain, because children may describe their knee as painful when the source of the pain is actually a problem in the hip, in the shaft of the bone above or below the knee, or even in the muscle. The most common example of this is a child with a slipped capital femoral epiphysis of the hip (see "Hip Pain," in this chapter). The child should have blood work that includes a complete blood count, a metabolic profile, and muscle enzymes. Other diagnostic tests that may be useful in pinpointing the problem include ultrasound, MRI, bone scan, and aspirating fluid from the knee to check for the presence of bacteria or blood (see Chapter 22).

Specific Knee Conditions

Osgood-Schlatter disease is the result of inflammation of the patellar tendon where it attaches to the lower leg. As children grow, it takes time for the tendons (tissues that attach muscle to bone) to become firmly attached to the bone. During periods of rapid development, such as from nine to fifteen years of age, children's muscles often strengthen more rapidly than the tendon-bone attachment does. Running and kicking, such as while playing sports, leads to repeated pulling on the tendon where it attaches to the bone, and the child develops inflammation at that spot. As a result, the anterior tibial tubercle (the bump just below the knee) becomes swollen and tender (Fig. 3-1).

The pain in Osgood-Schlatter disease is brought on by activity and relieved by rest. It is never associated with stiffness or swelling of the knee itself, only the bump below the knee. It does not cause pain when children wake up in the morning, and it does not wake children up from sleep. The key to diagnosing Osgood-Schlatter disease is to realize that the pain is not in the knee (although that is how the children usually describe it). On careful examination, the knee is entirely normal. The pain is reproduced by pressing on the anterior tibial tubercle (the prominent bump just below the knee). Most often the tenderness is present on both sides, but it may be only the dominant side (e.g., the right if the child is right-handed). The key to treatment is rest, so the inflamed tendon and

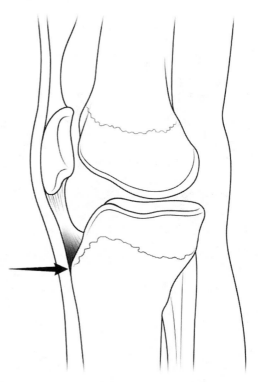

FIG 3-1 *Inflammation of the tendon insertion in Osgood-Schlatter's disease, producing pain just below the knee. The arrow indicates the anterior tibial tubercle.*

bone can heal and the tendon-bone attachment can become stronger and withstand the pulling by the muscles.

Sinding-Larsen-Johansson disease is similar in its cause to Osgood-Schlatter disease. This condition is common in the early teenage years as well as among teenagers who are doing a lot of jumping in sports such as basketball and volleyball. Jumping increases stress on the knee, with sudden pulling on the tendon that attaches to the bottom of the kneecap (patella). As a result, these children complain of knee pain whenever they jump. On examination, they have pain when the bottom of the kneecap is pressed (see Fig. 3-2). This condition should be treated by resting the knee and avoiding jumping activities. **Jumper's knee** is a more severe injury occurring in older children, though the mechanism of the injury is the same. In jumper's knee there is a deep tear of the tendon itself that may ultimately require surgery to relieve the pain.

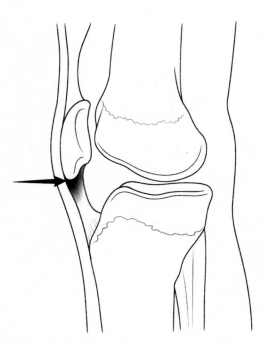

FIG 3-2 *Irritation where the tendon attaches to the bottom of the kneecap (patella) causes pain with jumping, which can be reproduced by pressing on the bottom of the patella in teenagers with Sinding-Larsen-Johansson disease.*

Chronic knee pain can be caused by a number of mechanical conditions that primarily result from excessive wear and tear on the knee and surrounding tissues. **Chondromalacia patella** or **patellofemoral dysfunction** causes knee pain that is much worse when going downhill or downstairs. Despite the large number of children and young adults who suffer from this condition, it is poorly understood. Although there are many proposed treatments for patellofemoral dysfunction, only two are generally agreed upon. The first is to avoid the activities that aggravate the condition. The second is a program of exercises that involve lifting the leg as it is held straight, which increases the strength of the muscles around the knee without bending it. **Osteochondritis dissecans** is the development of a dense area of damaged bone along the edge of the joint line. This may be the result of direct trauma or overuse. It is a common injury in children who have continued running and jumping activities despite pain. It may respond to extended immobilization, but in some cases the fragment of damaged bone will fall into the joint. If this happens, the knee may lock and surgery may be required to remove the fragment. Finally, **iliotibial band syndrome** can cause pain along the thigh and the outer edge of the knee. It is caused by tightening of a band of tissue that runs along the outside (lateral) edge of the leg and anchors to the knee. The pain comes on with running, but only after an extended period. It is often aggravated by climbing stairs, in contrast to chondromalacia patella, which is made worse by going downstairs. A program of stretching and leg-strengthening exercises is often sufficient to correct this problem.

Osteoid osteomas are benign tumors of the bone, much like knots in wood. Often they never cause difficulty. However, in some children they cause pain. Most often the pain occurs in the middle of the night and is sufficiently severe to wake the child. They occur in boys more often than girls and frequently become symptomatic during the teenage years. They are most common in the region of the hip (see "Hip Pain") but may occur either above or below the knee. Osteoid osteomas around the knee are usually easily diagnosed on routine X-rays, but sometimes a CAT scan is required to recognize them. The pain from an osteoid osteoma is usually easily relieved by acetaminophen or ibuprofen. All children in whom there is any possibility that the lesion may be a serious bone tumor and all children whose pain is not easily relieved by these medications require careful evaluation by an orthopedist with extensive experience in these lesions.

Plicae are folds of synovial tissue that may be seen in the knee on MRI. They are a normal finding and not usually a cause of pain. If a child has vague unexplained knee pains and a plica is noted on MRI, orthopedists may suggest arthroscopic surgery. However, there is a good chance that the plica is not the cause of the pain. Proper treatment of children with plicae centers on excluding other causes of the pain. Once that has been done, most children are advised to avoid the activities causing pain. If the pain persists despite these measures or the activity cannot be reasonably avoided, the family may wish to consider surgery. Since early arthritis is accompanied by thickening of the synovium, it is not rare for a child with arthritis to be misdiagnosed as having plicae.

Plant thorn synovitis is an arthritis that occurs in children who have fallen on a palm frond, cactus thorn, or similar piece of sharp plant material and a part of the plant has broken off inside the knee. The knee is usually red and hot with no history of injury. The key to recognizing plant thorn synovitis is a proper history. Usually the child lives someplace warm (e.g., Florida, the Caribbean, southern California) or traveled there several weeks before the problem started. The child is typically four to six years old—just old enough to get out of sight and fall down. He or she had a small cut on the knee that healed quickly. No one remembers this cut when the knee is hot and swollen weeks later. It is important to recognize plant thorn synovitis because it will not respond to antibiotics or nonsteroidal anti-inflammatory drugs (NSAIDs). Proper treatment requires a synovectomy (cleaning out all of the inflamed tissue lining the knee). When this is done, the diagnosis of plant thorn synovitis can be confirmed by looking at the tissue under polarized light. This will show starch granules from the plant material that broke off inside the knee.

Blount's disease refers to bowing of the legs (genu varum). Young children may develop Blount's disease without any apparent explanation. There is a sudden shift in growth of the tibia (the main bone in the lower leg) and the inner edge no longer grows as well as the outer edge. With progressive growth of the outer edge the legs are forced to bow. In small children, this is most often painless and it affects both sides. In teenagers, Blount's disease is often associated with obesity. In these children, it is suspected that the excessive weight puts too much stress on the inner side of the tibia and the growth plate is damaged. Under these circumstances, one side may be affected and not the other. Blount's disease in teenagers may be associated with progressive pain. At first the pain may be intermittent and relieved by acetaminophen or other pain relievers, but over time it may steadily worsen. If it is left untreated, the pain will continue and the damage to the joint may result in the premature development of mechanical arthritis. An orthopedic surgeon should monitor children of all ages with Blount's disease. Bracing and surgical intervention are sometimes necessary.

There are two types of infection that must be considered in a child with knee pain. **Septic arthritis** is an infection in the joint itself. **Osteomyelitis** is an infection in the bone. In the knee, osteomyelitis is more common than septic arthritis. Often osteomyelitis occurs near the ends of the bones and produces pain in the joint near the infected bone. The pain of osteomyelitis may wax and wane, but the child is never free of pain. In children with osteomyelitis, the pain usually gets steadily worse over a few days at most. These children often have fevers and look ill, but occasionally the child looks well and is only limping. If the infection has been present for a period of time, it should be easy to see on X-rays. However, during the first few days after an infection begins, the X-ray may not show changes. Bone scans and MRIs will demonstrate infections in the bone even at the earliest stages.

A **sympathetic effusion** has its cause elsewhere in the leg but produces symptoms in the knee. In this situation, there may be an infection or a tumor (even leukemia) in the bone. At the same time the child will complain of pain and have an obviously swollen knee. Aspiration of the knee will show fluid that suggests arthritis and not an infection. The key to suspecting this situation is that these children are in more pain than would be expected from arthritis. In addition, careful examination will indicate that they are very tender in the shaft of the bone, not just in the joint itself.

Unicameral bone cysts are large cystic malformations of the bone that may occur in the femur (also in the humerus, the bone of the upper arm). They usually are entirely asymptomatic unless there is a fracture, in which case the child should be cared for by an experienced orthopedist. Following healing of the fracture, the orthopedist may choose to treat the lesion by direct injections of corticosteroids or curettage. **Aneurismal bone cysts** differ in having a significant blood vessel component in the cyst. They tend to grow more rapidly than unicameral bone cysts and are more likely to be discovered because they are causing pain. Like unicameral bone cysts, they are easily found by routine X-ray. The majority of bone cysts are minor. However, because they can be associated with more serious problems, children with bone cysts should be referred to an experienced orthopedist for evaluation.

While many **bone tumors** are benign, some are malignant and life-threatening. A full discussion of the types of bone tumors and their treatment is far beyond the scope of this book, but like tumors elsewhere, bone tumors begin very small and grow relatively slowly. Often they are easily visible on routine X-ray by the time they are producing pain.

HIP PAIN

Most often, children with hip pain walk with a very abnormal gait. If the pain is sudden and severe, the child may not be able to walk at all. A child who is unable to walk after trauma or a fall needs immediate medical evaluation to exclude fractures and other orthopedic injuries. A child who wakes up in the morning with sudden hip pain and has difficulty walking may be suffering from any of a number of conditions. If the pain does not disappear after a few minutes, the child should be brought for immediate medical attention to exclude the possibility of an infection. All children with hip pain should receive a careful and thorough medical evaluation, including children with pain that disappears after a few minutes but keeps coming back.

Often pain in the hip is in fact pain in various parts of the pelvis. With excessive physical activity it is common to develop pain where muscles attach to the pelvis. Children with chronic hip injuries typically report pain with certain movements and activities, and the pain is relieved by rest. However, the hip is a deep-seated joint, and injuries such as ligamentous tears are infrequent in childhood.

Specific Hip Conditions

Toxic synovitis is an inflammation of the hip that typically occurs in children from four to six years of age. Although it often occurs in children with evidence of a viral respiratory infection, its cause is unknown. Children with toxic synovitis have a very characteristic story. Most often the child went to bed well or with a slight sniffle the night before. In the morning the child has severe hip pain and is unable to walk. Because the symptoms are so dramatic, the children are immediately brought to the doctor. Often there is a low-grade fever and blood tests may show an elevated white blood cell count and slight elevation of the erythrocyte sedimentation rate. The immediate concern is to exclude a bacterial infection of the hip, which can worsen dramatically over a period of only a few hours, and so these children are often referred to an orthopedist, who may remove fluid from the hip to look for signs of infection. In contrast, I have often seen children with toxic synovitis who are already improving by the time they reach my office. Ultrasound is increasingly being used to differentiate bacterial infection from toxic synovitis. However, if there is any doubt, aspiration of fluid from the hip, hospitalization, and antibiotic therapy are appropriate until the possibility of an infection has been excluded.

Once the diagnosis of toxic synovitis has been made, children may be treated with NSAIDs and rest. They usually recover completely within a few days, though there may be some residual irritability of the hip for several weeks. The prognosis for these children is very good.

A diagnosis of recurrent toxic synovitis should be regarded with suspicion, since true toxic synovitis is not a recurrent condition. Some children have Legg-Calve-Perthes disease (see below) that has not been recognized. In other children, recurrent episodes of synovitis in the hip may be the first manifestation of what will ultimately become obvious spondyloarthropathy. Any child diagnosed with recurrent synovitis should have a thorough evaluation by a pediatric rheumatologist if possible. Also, toxic synovitis should never be diagnosed in a child over nine years of age, in whom isolated synovitis of the hip is usually the initial manifestation of a spondyloarthropathy (though other causes of hip inflammation must be excluded).

Legg-Calve-Perthes disease (LCP) results from softening of the head of the femur (the long bone of the leg), which gradually becomes distorted and may flatten or crumble (see Fig. 3-3). It is thought that this results from problems with the blood supply to the head of the femur, which may be caused by an injury or congenital abnormality. One report has suggested that LCP occurs far more frequently in the children of parents who smoke. However, problems with the environment or blood supply cannot be the whole answer, since LCP occurs four times more often in boys than in girls.

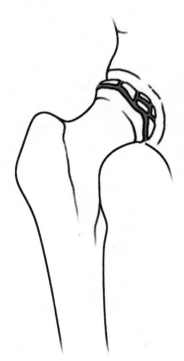

LCP usually begins in young children (commonly four to six years of age), who are most often noticed to be limping before there is any complaint of pain. Over time, the limp becomes more noticeable and the child may begin to complain of pain. At the earliest stages an MRI may be required to diagnose LCP. However, if the symptoms have been present for more than several weeks, it should be possible to make the diagnosis with a regular X-ray of the hip. This will show flattening of the head of the femur. Most cases of LCP involve only one hip, but in a few children both hips are involved. Premature birth and problems during the newborn period increase the risk of LCP, as does a family history of the disease.

FIG 3-3 *Changes in the head of the femur resulting from Legg-Calve-Perthes disease.*

Children diagnosed with LCP should be under the care of an orthopedist. Treatment often consists initially of traction followed by casting. Once the cast is removed, physical therapy is important to restore strength and range of motion. The purpose of the traction and casting is to keep the femur properly seated in the hip while decreasing the pressure on the femoral head. Often this allows the bone to reestablish its blood supply and begin to repair itself. The precise details of treatment will depend on the age of the child and the degree of damage to the bone at the time the problem is discovered.

Children with bilateral LCP should be thoroughly evaluated. In some instances, this is a sign of an underlying condition such as hyperthyroidism or sickle-cell disease. In others, the deformed head of the femur may be the result of more widespread conditions, such as multiple epiphyseal dysplasia or spondyloepiphyseal dysplasia tarda. These orthopedic conditions are recognized by the presence of abnormal epiphyses (the ends of the bone that insert into the joints) in multiple joints, as seen on a complete set of X-rays. The long-term prognosis for children with LCP who are diagnosed early is good. If the disease has been present for a long time, the bone may already have begun healing itself by the time the disease is recognized. In many children, this healing is adequate and things go well. However, in some children, there may be permanent damage to the bone. There is also concern that children with residual damage from LCP may have persistent mechanical problems that will cause them to have mechanical arthritis of the hip, leading to problems when they become adults.

Sickle-cell anemia may cause pain in the bones because of blood vessels being blocked by abnormally shaped red blood cells. This may occur in the blood vessels that supply the hip and result in damage to the femur. When it does, it looks exactly like—and essentially is—LCP. In children with severe sickle-cell anemia, other bones may be damaged also and there may be widespread joint problems. Usually a child with these problems will have been recognized to have sickle-cell disease long before the bone problems begin.

There are two basic types of infections that must be considered in children with hip pain. **Septic arthritis** is an infection in the joint itself, whereas **osteomyelitis** is an infection in the bone. In the hip, septic arthritis is more common than osteomyelitis.

For many years *Haemophilus influenzae* was the bacterium responsible for most septic infections of the hip, but now most children are vaccinated against this infection and it has become rare. Staphylococcal and streptococcal infections of the hip do still occur. It is also possible to have a tuberculosis infection in the hip. At present, Lyme disease may be the most common cause of infectious arthritis involving the hip for people living in endemic areas of the United States (see Chapter 8).

Most infections in the hip are sudden in onset and associated with rapidly worsening symptoms of pain, fever, and difficulty in walking. A child with these symptoms should be seen by a physician as soon as possible. Tuberculosis may cause slowly worsening symptoms of hip pain. A child with an acutely painful hip should be seen by an orthopedist. Although there may be some initial confusion between children with infections and those with toxic synovitis, children with toxic synovitis usually improve rapidly without treatment. If there is serious concern that the joint may be infected, it should be aspirated for appropriate studies, including bacterial cultures. Chronic hip pain associated with stiffness is more likely to be the result of enthesitis-associated arthritis involving the hip (see Chapter 7), but the possibility of an infection should always be given careful consideration.

Osteomyelitis often occurs near the ends of the bones and produces pain in the joint near the infection. The pain of osteomyelitis may wax and wane, but the child is never free of pain and the pain usually gets steadily worse over a period of a few days. Children with osteomyelitis often have fevers and look ill, but occasionally the child looks well and is only limping. If the infection has been present for more than a few days, it should be easy to detect on X-rays. However, during the first few days after an infection begins, the X-ray may not show changes. Bone scans and MRIs will demonstrate infections in the bone at the earliest stages when pain is present.

Pain in the lower abdomen near the hip may be a cause of confusion. When dealing with younger children, it can be difficult to know exactly where the pain is coming from. Children with severe lower abdominal pain may walk with an abnormal gait, suggesting arthritis or an infected hip. A ruptured appendix should always be considered in children with pain in the right side of the pelvis without an obvious explanation.

Osteoid osteomas are benign tumors of the bone. See the section on these tumors under "Knee Pain," above.

Slipped capital femoral epiphysis (SCFE) is an injury to the growth plate of the femur (the bone in the upper leg) that results in the epiphysis, the growing end of the bone, slipping off the shaft (see Fig. 3-4). This injury occurs most

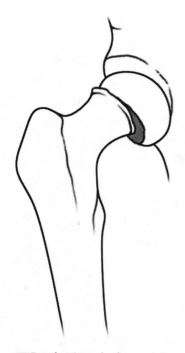

FIG 3-4 *This is the characteristic appearance of a slipped capital femoral epiphysis. The epiphysis is the rounded portion of the bone in the hip joint. It has literally slipped off the end of the long bone (femur). Compare this with Fig. 3-3, where the epiphysis has crumbled but remains in the proper position.*

often in boys between the ages of ten and fifteen years but may occur in girls and occasionally is seen in younger children. It occurs more often in African Americans and in children who are overweight. The most dramatic cases of SCFE occur as an injury with sudden slipping of the epiphysis. This produces acute hip pain and inability to walk. X-rays to confirm the diagnosis should include both standard views and "frog leg" views in which the child is instructed to bend the knees and spread them apart. SCFE may be missed on standard views of the hips, but the slippage is usually obvious on the "frog leg" views.

Some children develop SCFE on a more gradual basis. No one is sure why this happens. These children will have progressive onset of pain and stiffness in the involved hip. SCFE may also occur in children with hypothyroidism and other growth problems. In about one-third of children, the disease is bilateral. The slip on the opposite side may be present when the first SCFE is noted or may occur later.

Because deep pain may be difficult to localize, the child may describe the pain as coming from the groin, the thigh, or the knee instead of the hip. Children with a chronic slip usually have an obvious limp. The changes in the bone may force the hip on the affected side to rotate outward. The abnormal alignment of the bones that results triggers muscle spasm. This muscle spasm causes children with chronic SCFE to report stiffness with rest and increased pain with activity, symptoms that suggest arthritis. The chronic slippage should be evident on X-ray. In uncertain or difficult cases, an MRI may be useful to confirm the diagnosis.

Orthopedists treat SCFE by putting a pin in the bone to hold the epiphysis in place while the bone heals. If detected and treated early, children with SCFE usually do well. Chronic SCFE that is not promptly treated may result in damage to the head of the hip bone (femur). This can result in a permanent limp, difference in the length of the two legs, and early onset of arthritis due to mechanical damage.

Iliotibial band syndrome, discussed above under "Knee Pain," may also produce pain at the hip. In these cases, children typically complain of a snapping sensation with certain movements. Often this is associated with trochanteric bursitis (see Fig. 3-5 and the next section), which may be the result of excessive activity. Iliotibial band syndrome may also occur in children with a spondyloarthropathy (see Chapter 7). Iliotibial band syndrome itself is a benign condition that does not normally require therapy. However, if the snapping is associated with a sensation of pain, further evaluation is warranted.

The greater trochanter is the large bump that sticks out on the side of the femur where it turns toward the knee. Because this protrusion is just under the skin at the side of the hip, it is protected by a bursa. The bursa is a small sac of fluid that allows easy movement of the tissues over the bone (see Fig. 3-5). With excessive running or other activities, this bursa may become inflamed, a condition called **trochanteric bursitis**. Typically, this is a problem of teenagers or adults and not younger children. The classic complaint is pain along the side of the leg that can be reproduced by pressure over the greater trochanter. The pain

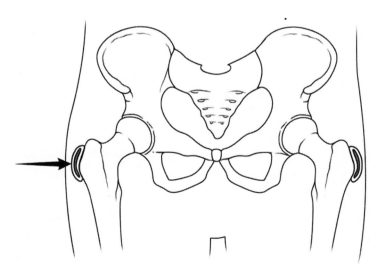

FIG 3-5 *Trochanteric bursitis results from irritation in the fluid-filled sacs (bursas) that are located just under the skin and over the greater trochanter.*

often is described as moving both up and down the side of the leg. Trochanteric bursitis is treated with ice, stretching exercises, and in more severe cases NSAIDs. In rare cases, children require injection of steroids into the bursa for relief.

The hip and pelvis may be the site of **avulsion fractures**, in which a tendon pulls off its attachment to the bone. These injuries are usually associated with the sensation of a snap or pop and immediate pain. X-rays typically confirm the diagnosis. **Stress fractures** in the femur or pelvis may come on more slowly. Children who participate in athletics may complain of progressively increasing groin pain with activities. Although stress fractures in the femur are not always evident on X-rays, most often they are obvious on bone scan. MRIs may also be helpful to confirm the diagnosis.

Congenital hip dislocation results from improper formation of the acetabulum, the socket on the pelvis into which the head of the hip bone inserts. This condition should be diagnosed in early childhood. Often it is first suspected when the pediatrician notices a "hip click" in the nursery. This is a sensation of clicking when the hip is moved in what is called the Ortolani maneuver. In most children, the hip click will go away after a period of observation and perhaps "double diapering" (the bulk of an extra diaper forces the legs into a frog leg position, which helps keep the head of the femur properly positioned). However, if it persists, orthopedic evaluation is needed.

Children with congenital hip dislocation walk with a waddling gait that is obvious to a trained observer but may be overlooked by parents. If the hip dislocation is present on only one side, it may be suspected when the parents or physician notice that the line under the curve of the buttock is not in the same position on both sides (asymmetric gluteal folds). The child will have decreased range of motion of the hips and abnormal X-rays. However, because the condition has always been there, the child may never have complained of pain.

Congenital hip dislocation is easily diagnosed if appropriate X-rays are done. It is treated by orthopedists. Cases detected in early life can often be managed without surgery. However, in severe cases surgical correction is necessary. If it is not detected and corrected, the hips may become severely damaged because of mechanical damage leading to degenerative arthritis. It is important that any child who walks with a waddling gait be appropriately evaluated.

The hip joint is rarely the first joint involved in children with **juvenile arthritis** (see Chapter 5), but it may become involved over time. In contrast, the hip is commonly the first joint involved in children with spondyloarthropathies (Chapter 7). These children often begin with complaints of stiffness in the hip or lower back when they wake up in the morning. Over time, they develop symptoms in other joints. However, they often have to be asked about and examined carefully for evidence of pain or limitation in the back, wrists, knees, or ankles, as they will not associate the complaints in other joints with their hip pain. Since spondyloarthropathies rarely begin in children before the age of ten, younger children with hip pain must be carefully evaluated to exclude other causes.

Mechanical arthritis may occur in children who have had damage to the bones of the hip from SCFE, congenital hip dislocation, or previous infection. These conditions and the mechanical cause of the arthritis are often evident on routine X-rays. If the routine X-rays do not provide an explanation for the pain, an MRI may be necessary.

Some children with **muscle or systemic diseases** will experience significant pain in the muscles in the front of the thigh. This pain may be mistakenly reported as coming from the hip or the knee (and in fact, hip and knee problems may cause pain in those muscles). Whenever a child complains of chronic pain and disability without obvious findings in the bones or joints, a careful evaluation for muscle or systemic diseases should be performed, including blood tests to measure muscle enzymes, thyroid function studies, a complete blood count, and appropriate MRIs and X-rays.

Unicameral bone cysts are large cystic malformations of the bone that may occur in the femur or the humerus. They usually do not produce any symptoms unless there is a fracture. Like bone cysts near the knee, they should be cared for by an experienced orthopedist. **Bone tumors** should be considered in the evaluation of children who initially have pain in the hip as well.

BACK PAIN

In this age of increasingly large book bags and backpacks, backache is becoming a more common complaint among adolescents. Fortunately, serious back problems remain uncommon. As is true for other regions of the body, the key to assisting the physician in properly diagnosing the cause of your child's back pain is the information you provide. When you take your child to be evaluated, you should be prepared to provide answers to the following questions:

- Did the pain come on suddenly following an injury or fall? Or slowly, over a period of days, without an injury?
- Does the pain wake the child up at night?
- Is the pain associated with stiffness and worse when the child first gets up in the morning? Or does the pain begin only with activities?
- Is the pain relieved by rest? Or does the child stiffen up if he or she sits for a long period?
- What position or activity makes the pain better? What makes it worse?
- Is the pain confined to a single location or does it move up and down the back?
- Does the pain extend down into one leg or out into one shoulder?

Serious back injuries are typically associated with severe trauma, such as accidents, falls, and sports injuries, and will not be covered here. True backaches not associated with injuries are rare in childhood. Structural abnormalities are the most common cause. Back pain due to structural abnormalities is extremely unusual before the age of ten years. Any young child complaining of back pain requires careful evaluation. Infections and tumors are serious causes of back pain that may be present in this age group. In older children, scoliosis and spondylolisthesis are the most common structural abnormalities that cause back pain. Usually they begin without symptoms, but over time compensatory changes occur that often cause mechanical pain.

Specific Conditions

Scoliosis is an abnormal curvature of the spine with rotation of the vertebrae. This curvature often results in one shoulder appearing higher than the other or the hips appearing uneven. Since the curvature occurs with growth, it is rare for scoliosis to become evident before the age of ten years. Once detected, it should be carefully evaluated and followed. Many children have only mild curvatures and require no treatment, but others have progressive disease requiring bracing and, less frequently, surgery. Scoliosis is usually painless and detected only on examination. Pain suggests that the scoliosis has been present for a prolonged period with secondary mechanical problems.

Children are routinely screened for scoliosis at school, but the expertise and thoroughness of the examiners vary widely. Most scoliosis is idiopathic (unexplained). In rare cases, scoliosis may be the result of tumors, infections, or damage to the spinal cord. These cases may appear at an earlier age than idiopathic scoliosis and be more severe. Any child whose spine appears crooked or has an abnormal scoliosis screening should have an orthopedic evaluation.

It is easy to examine a child for scoliosis. Have the child stand in front of you with both feet together and the heels lined up with each other. Then have the child bend forward to touch the toes. Two findings suggest scoliosis. The most common is a "rib hump," which means that the ribs on one side stick up higher than the ribs on the other (Fig. 3-6). In some children, there is a prominent low back (lumbar) component that is easily felt by putting your hand on the lower part of the back. If one side of the back is lower than the other, further evaluation by an orthopedist is necessary.

Spondylolisthesis is the slippage of one vertebra over another. Most often this occurs at the junction of the lumbar and sacral spine. Some cases may be due to a congenital weakness, while other cases may be due to poor healing after an injury. Either cause results in weakness of the bone bridges (posterior elements) that hold the spine in place. Spondylolisthesis results when this weakness allows one bone segment to slide forward over another. Although mild degrees of spondylolisthesis may be asymptomatic, more severe involvement characteristically leads to low back pain that may radiate down the back of the

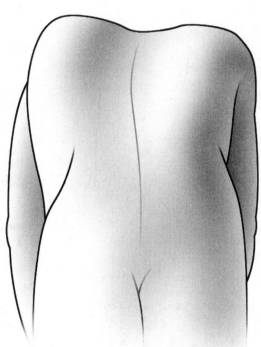

FIG 3-6 *A positive scoliosis screen, with the ribs on the left side appearing higher than the right when the child bends over. The shoulders may also appear uneven when the child is standing up, but this is more difficult to notice.*

thighs. Most children with this condition can be followed conservatively, but some require orthopedic intervention. Because the symptoms can worsen over time, all children with chronic back pain should be followed by an experienced orthopedist.

Some children have **kyphosis**, excessive curvature of the spine in which the spine is bent forward. If you look at the child from the side, you will see that the upper part of the back angles forward sharply (see Fig. 3-7). This abnormal forward curvature may be the result of abnormalities in the bone resulting from fractures or infections. However, most often it occurs without explanation. In severe cases the child may appear to have a hunchback.

Some children have postural kyphosis. This is usually a mild increase in the forward bend of the spine, leading to the appearance that they are always slumping over. These children often have no abnormal findings on X-ray. However, all children with this type of spinal curvature need to be investigated by an orthopedist with appropriate X-rays to find out why they have kyphosis. For children without significant abnormality, a program of exercises is often adequate.

A common cause of kyphosis in teenagers is **Scheuermann's disease**, thought to result from abnormalities in the growth of the vertebrae. This results in the front of the vertebrae being compressed relative to the back (see Fig. 3-7). The diagnosis is easily made with X-rays. Children with this condition may need to wear a brace to relieve their pain and prevent worsening of their condition. More severe or worsening cases may require orthopedic surgery.

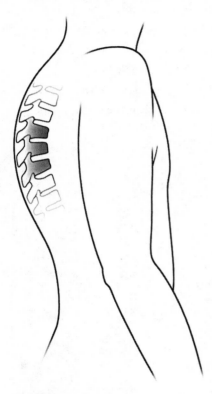

FIG 3-7 *Appearance of the spine with wedge-shaped vertebrae in a child with kyphosis due to Scheuermann's disease.*

Kyphosis may also be the result of damage to the bones of the spine by an infection, tumor, or poor bone formation. These conditions are all rare. Children with conditions that are known to damage the spine should be carefully monitored. Parents of children with poor bone formation or children who are taking medications that can damage the bones need to be reminded that their children should be watched carefully for spine problems. If a child has been diagnosed with an infection or a tumor in or around the spine, the family should be aware of the need to monitor the spine as the child grows.

There are a variety of **infections** that may damage the spine. Fortunately, none of them is common in childhood. Staphylococcal bacteria are common causes of infections that may affect the bones of the spine. Tuberculosis can also affect the bones of the spine (in which case it is sometimes called Potts' disease). Bacterial infections of the spine are usually very painful. They are easily diagnosed by either X-rays or bone scans (Chapter 22). Despite many claims to the contrary, back pain in children is not a result of Lyme disease.

Discitis is a confusing cause of back pain in younger children. Typically, it affects children under the age of ten. These children may have initial symptoms of a cold or flu-like illness. They then develop severe back pain, but in this age group they may not be able to describe it. The key to recognizing this illness in very young children is that they suddenly refuse to sit up or walk. The cause of discitis remains unclear. In some cases, a bacterium such as staphylococcus is identified and the infection is treated with antibiotics, but often no causative bacterium can be identified. This illness is usually diagnosed on the basis of the typical clinical picture with a bone scan and MRI or X-rays to be sure that no other problem is present.

The benign bone tumors called **osteoid osteomas** are a cause of chronic low-grade bone pain that may occur in many different locations. (See the discussion under "Knee Pain" in this chapter.) Osteoid osteomas in the spine typically come to parents' attention when a child complains of chronic back pain that comes and goes without explanation. A typical child with an osteoid osteoma reports a sense of deep aching pain, often worse at night. Untreated painful osteoid osteomas may cause major problems because the pain causes muscle spasms.

A fairly common cause of chronic back pain in adolescents is **spondylolysis**. This is a stress fracture of the pars interarticularis (see Fig. 3-8). It is often the result of excessive stress on the low back from dancing, running, weight lifting, or other activities. Female participants in gymnastics are prone to this injury. As with stress fractures in other locations, the complaint of pain is usually exacerbated by activity and relieved by rest. X-rays may reveal the fracture, but in some cases an MRI or bone scan may be required. Children with this type of pain

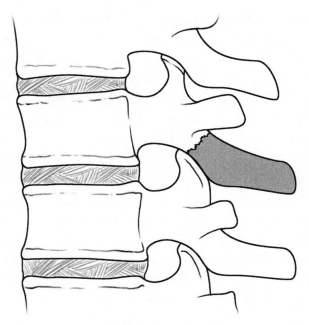

FIG 3-8 *Stress fracture of the pars interarticularis (darkened segment), causing back pain.*

should be carefully questioned about pain in other joints or stiffness when they arise in the morning, as these symptoms may indicate arthritis.

A common complaint among adults, **disc herniation** is usually the result of an excessive stress put on the spine with the resultant rupture of the cushioning material in one of the intervertebral discs. This condition is quite rare in children, though you can check for this by having the child lie on his or her back and raise one leg while keeping it straight (see Fig. 3-9). A child who has pain during this maneuver may have significant disc herniation and should be promptly evaluated.

Although an MRI of the spine is very accurate at identifying disc problems, finding minor disc problems on the MRI is not a reliable explanation for back pain; many individuals who do not experience back pain have minor disc herniation on an MRI. Although it is not impossible for a teenager to have a damaged disc, parents should be extremely skeptical about this diagnosis as the cause of back pain. Gradual onset of back pain with stiffness on awakening is more likely to be associated with a spondyloarthropathy or other illness.

Low back pain and morning stiffness are commonly due to spondyloarthropathies in teenagers. However, adolescents rarely come to the doctor complaining

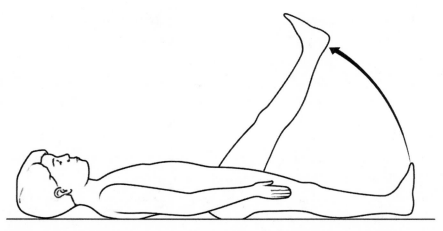

FIG 3-9 *Any child with pain when the straight leg is raised while lying flat on the back requires prompt medical evaluation.*

of low back pain when they wake up in the morning. Since the onset is very gradual, most accept this stiffness as normal. The key to suspecting a spondyloarthropathy as the cause of an adolescent's back pain lies in carefully examining the teenager and finding evidence of arthritis or tendon insertion pain (enthesitis) elsewhere. A strong family history of back pain also should suggest this diagnosis. A key indication is that children with spondyloarthropathies almost never can bend over and touch their toes. See Chapter 7 for more information.

NECK PAIN

Neck pain in children is rare. Most often it is due to muscle irritation involving the muscles that hold the head and shoulders in the proper position. Frequently this is because of a heavy backpack improperly carried over just one shoulder, which places unnecessary strain on the muscles.

Before you go to the physician's office with your child's complaints of neck pain, think about the answers to the questions at the beginning of the section on back pain. Since the neck is simply the top portion of the back, the same questions need to be asked about complaints here. Several additional questions should also be asked.

- Is the child having headaches? Do they occur at the same time as the neck pain?

- Is the child having jaw pain? Spasm in the muscles around the jaw may be reported as neck pain.
- Is the child having problems seeing?
- What type of pillow does the child use?

Specific Conditions

In **wryneck**, also called torticollis, the child holds the head to one side because of problems with the sternocleidomastoid muscle, at the front of the neck. This muscle is sometimes injured at birth and becomes shortened as a result of the injury. Children with this problem may develop neck pain as they get older and their muscles try to compensate. Wryneck in older children is usually due to an injury to a neck muscle, such as from carrying a heavy backpack on one side.

Neck muscle injury is the most common cause of neck pain in children. If the pain is severe, there may be muscle spasm, forcing the child to hold the head tilted to one side for comfort. Pain due to irritation of the sternocleidomastoid muscle radiates into the front of the chest. In contrast, pain due to irritation of the trapezius muscle radiates down into the middle of the back and out toward the shoulder on the affected side. The child may go to bed at night without complaint but wake up the next day stiff and sore, unable to straighten the neck.

The muscles of the neck may also become inflamed by severe sore throat, resulting from infections in the tonsils and infections or other causes of irritation elsewhere in the nose and throat. Similar problems may result from irritation of the jaw, producing spasm of the muscles where the neck and jaw meet. Any child in whom this is a persistent problem without explanation should be evaluated by an ear, nose, and throat specialist (otolaryngologist).

There are congenital bone problems that affect the neck, such as **Klippel-Feil syndrome**. These are easily diagnosed on X-ray. Other bone problems such as **osteoid osteoma** (see "Knee Pain") may occur in the neck with findings identical to when they occur lower in the back. Herniated discs (see "Back Pain") and infections may also occur in the neck. It is important to recognize that these problems may initially be reported as headaches and not recognized as coming from the neck.

While **spondyloarthropathies** predominantly affect the low back, in some children they cause neck pain. In most but not all cases, these children will have previously been recognized to have involvement of multiple joints.

Certain forms of juvenile arthritis commonly lead to problems with the bones in the neck. These children have limited neck motion (often they cannot look up or down or turn their heads from side to side without moving their backs). In some cases, this loss of motion is associated with pain, but more often it occurs gradually and the patient is not immediately aware of the problem.

Any child with prolonged, severe, or unexplained neck pain should be thoroughly investigated with a complete physical examination. If the problem is persistent and the answer has not been found, consideration should be given to evaluation by a neurologist, an ear, nose, and throat specialist, a neurosurgeon or orthopedist who deals with neck problems, and a rheumatologist.

LOWER LEG, FOOT, ANKLE, HEEL, AND TOE PAIN

Each area of the foot has a different set of common problems and solutions, so you need to be able to tell the physician where the pain is. You can both ask the child to point and examine the child's foot yourself to see whether any part of the foot is red, swollen, or tender.

There are some very knowledgeable podiatrists, but children should be thoroughly evaluated by an orthopedist and, if appropriate, a rheumatologist before being referred to a podiatrist.

Lower Leg Pain

Shin splints are a common complaint of children who do a lot of running. They typically occur in children who are trying to do too much too fast. Often the problem disappears with additional conditioning. Children with continuing pain in the shin area (tibia) should be evaluated with X-rays to be sure there is not a more serious problem (stress fractures, infections, etc.). Arch supports and orthotics may be helpful in chronic cases.

Chronic compartment syndrome may be a cause of calf pain in very active children. These children often feel well but complain of pain in the calf region after being active for a significant period. The pain disappears with rest but recurs with activity. Often these children complain of tenderness when the calf is squeezed. Typically, the problem is one-sided and occurs in the dominant leg (i.e., the right leg if the child is right-handed). The pain results from enlargement of the muscles with exercise to the point where they are constricted by the surrounding tissues. If the problem does not resolve with a period of rest, surgery may be required.

Toe Pain

In a young child, toe pain is often a source of confusion because the child cannot reliably tell you what happened. When a child points to one toe and says it hurts, we all start by thinking that it was banged, got stepped on, or is being pinched in a shoe. Real trauma to the toe is usually obvious. The toe is very painful and there is often a bruise. Whenever this occurs, the foot should be X-rayed to make sure nothing is broken. With the exception of fractures, minor trauma to the toe should be better in a day or two.

When the toe has been injured, there is often discoloration under the toenail. If there is no discoloration and the pain persists, you should compare it to the same toe on the other foot. If it is very red and swollen, it may be infected and should be evaluated by a physician immediately. If the toe on one side looks bigger than the one on the other but the child is not complaining, squeeze it gently. Often the toe is tender and the child will pull the foot away. If that happens, gently take the foot in your hand and squeeze just behind where the toe attaches to the foot. If that is also tender, it suggests arthritis.

Pain due to bleeding under the toenail, known as **tennis toe**, is most commonly an injury in older children but may occur in younger children whose shoes are too small. It is the result of the toes forcibly colliding with the front of the shoe during activities. The acute pain can be relieved by allowing the blood to escape from under the toenail, which releases the pressure (this can be done by a physician).

The most common cause for **ingrown toenails** in children is nails that are cut too short, so the nail grows under the skin in front of it. Most often, ingrown toenails can be treated with warm soaks and local antibiotic creams, but this can be an extremely painful condition and may be associated with serious infections. Severe cases may require antibiotics and surgical removal of the offending toenail.

Freiberg's infarct, found in older children, is a degeneration of the end of the metatarsal bones (the long bones in the foot that extend to the base of the toes). Freiberg's infarct most often occurs in girls and usually at the base of the second toe. It is easily diagnosed if the appropriate X-rays are taken. It is treated with casting and use of an orthotic device to relieve the pressure placed on that portion of the foot. This condition may occur in other toes but rarely if ever involves the small toe.

Children complaining of pain at the base of the toes should be carefully examined for problems in other joints, which may indicate arthritis.

Heel Pain

Direct trauma to the heel is rare. It may occur if the foot is stepped on or if something falls on it. These injuries are obvious. Injuries to the heel may also occur with landing wrong after jumping, but again the injury is immediately evident.

Chronic heel pain associated with increased physical activity in preteens may be **Sever's disease**. In this condition, the heel bone is often tender to pressure and the heel cords may be tight. Some physicians will make this diagnosis based on X-rays showing irregularity and increased density of a portion of the bone behind the heel bone (sclerosis of the calcaneal apophysis). This is incorrect, as identical changes are commonly found on X-rays of children without foot pain. Sever's disease is not associated with pain in the tendons above or below the heel. Heel pain accompanied by pain in these tendons is often a sign of a spondyloarthropathy (Chapter 7).

Isolated **plantar fasciitis** (pain at the bottom of the heel where the tendons from the front of the foot attach) and **Achilles tendonitis** (pain at the back of the heel where the tendons coming down from the calf muscles attach) occur as overuse injuries in runners and other athletes. Since these findings may also be part of spondyloarthropathy, the key to proper diagnosis is a careful history and physical examination. Often a child with recurrent ankle sprains turns out to have back stiffness and hip limitation too, all of which are indicative of spondyloarthropathy.

Midfoot Pain

A number of different conditions may cause pain in the middle of the foot. Again, acute injuries are obvious and easily recognized with appropriate X-rays. The most common serious cause of chronic foot pain in active children is a **stress fracture of the metatarsals**. Stress fractures are overuse injuries found in many different sports, ranging from football and soccer to dance and gymnastics, and can occur in other parts of the body as well. They are typically treated with casting and rest. Although the initial X-ray may not show the fracture, follow-up X-rays should demonstrate healing bone to confirm the diagnosis.

Chronic pain in the middle of the foot is often the result of a variety of bony abnormalities. The most common of these is **flat feet**. Painless flat feet are most often a variation of normal and require no treatment. However, if a child with flat feet has foot pain, it requires evaluation. Often no significant abnormality is found and the pain is relieved with the use of an orthotic.

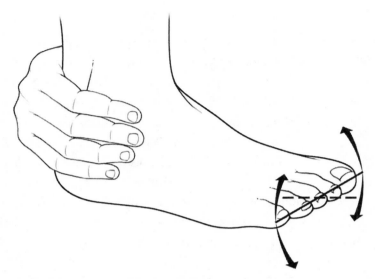

FIG 3-10 *Twisting the front of the foot while holding the heel steady. This is how to evaluate for the possibility of a rigid flat foot. The front of the foot should twist easily.*

Some children have a "rigid" flat foot. This is easy to recognize because it is difficult to move the different parts of the child's foot in relation to each other. Normally you should be able to simply hold the child's foot in your hand and turn the front part in different directions while holding the heel steady (see Fig. 3-10). In children with a rigid flat foot, it is necessary to determine whether the rigidity is being caused by **tarsal coalition** (fibrous bands between two or more of the bones in the middle of the foot that restrict motion and thus reduce flexibility) or another abnormality that can be corrected with casting or surgery. Every child with a rigid flat foot should be evaluated by an orthopedist.

An **accessory tarsal navicular bone** is an extra little piece of bone that forms at the base of the navicular bone in the midfoot. The extra bone is easily seen on X-ray. This extra piece of bone sticks out on the inside of the foot and may be painful and tender where it rubs against the inside of the shoe. Many people have these and never realize it. Stretching the shoe or wearing wider shoes often will eliminate the problem. Rare cases may require surgery. Occasionally the extra piece of bone leads to a mistaken diagnosis of a fracture.

Kohler's disease is an irregularity of the navicular bone, located in the middle of the foot, behind the metatarsal of the big toe. A typical patient with Kohler's disease is a child under the age of ten who complains of pain when walking and tenderness when the bone is pressed. It can be diagnosed by X-rays or a CAT scan. Kohler's disease usually resolves without treatment, but severe or persistent cases are often treated by casting.

Bunions are commonly thought of as a disease of adults. However, they may occur in teenagers, girls more often than boys. With activity these bunions may cause pain. Treatment usually centers on finding properly fitting shoes and other conservative measures. Surgery is generally unnecessary.

Pes cavus refers to a condition in which the arch of the foot is unusually high. Children with this uncommon condition often complain of foot pain when running. Usually both feet are affected equally. If only one side is affected, there is often a neurologic problem. Even when both sides are affected, there may be an underlying neuromuscular condition. All children with pes cavus should be carefully examined by an orthopedic specialist. Surgery to correct the deformity may be necessary.

Arthritis involving the subtalar joint may occur as a complication of many different forms of childhood arthritis. (The talus is the major bone in the foot where it connects to the leg at the ankle joint. The subtalar joint is located in the middle of the foot, where this bone connects to the bones of the front of the foot.) Because the subtalar joint is responsible for twisting movements of the foot, children with arthritis of the subtalar joint experience pain and difficulty walking on uneven surfaces. Subtalar joint involvement is just one part of a much larger picture in children with arthritis. It may be treated with NSAIDs or local injection. Some children with persistent pain benefit from the use of orthotics that prevent motion in the subtalar joint by holding the foot in a rigid position inside the shoe.

Diffuse foot pain is infrequent. One of the most common causes is **reflex sympathetic dystrophy**, which may begin after an injury to the foot. Children with reflex sympathetic dystrophy often experience color changes in the foot accompanied by profound hypersensitivity. Many of these children cannot put on a shoe or even a sock. This is a complex condition requiring specialized treatment; see Chapter 18.

Ankle Pain

The ankle is particularly vulnerable in growing children. Most ankle sprains are easily recognized and treated. More severe injuries should be evaluated by a physician to determine whether X-rays are necessary to exclude the possibility of a fracture. This is especially true if there is evidence of bruising. Chronic or recurrent ankle injuries require careful medical evaluation. Some of these are due to partial tears of the ligaments that support the ankle. Others may be due to damage to the growth plates of the bones.

A child with recurrent ankle pain without obvious injury should be investigated fully. Some children with recurrent ankle sprains in fact have inflamed tendons (enthesitis) from arthritis. Children with enthesitis-associated arthritis may have marked tendon swelling and tenderness, especially around the ankle. On careful examination, many of these children have enthesitis around multiple joints that has been overlooked. With appropriate diagnosis and treatment, they are often able to resume full activity.

ELBOW, SHOULDER, WRIST, AND FINGER PAIN

Pain in the fingers, wrists, elbows, and shoulders is common in older adults. But in young children, complaints are infrequent. Most complaints of pain in children under the age of ten are associated with minor injuries. Over the age of ten, overuse with athletic competition becomes more of an issue.

Elbow Pain

Nursemaid's elbow is one of the more common causes of distress in young children. Parents usually notice that a young child (two to three years is the peak age group) is holding the arm bent and not using it. It is most often the left arm, but either may be involved. Typically, the injury occurs when a parent or sibling tugs hard on the arm as the child is leaning away. It can also happen if you pick the child up by the arm (this should be avoided). The excessive stress on the elbow causes the bones to shift out of position, or dislocate. As a result, the child has pain and cannot straighten the arm. Commonly, the dislocated elbow will snap back into place by itself, but if not, an experienced physician can usually snap the elbow back into place by holding the elbow steady and rotating the thumb toward the middle of the body.

A physician should evaluate children complaining of continuing elbow pain because there may be an associated fracture or other problems requiring correction. Elbow fractures are not always easily seen on X-rays. Although isolated episodes of nursemaid's elbow are not uncommon, repeated or prolonged dislocations of the elbow may lead to permanent damage.

Trips and falls are the major cause of pain in the hand or wrist. Serious fractures are unusual without major trauma, but **greenstick** or **buckle fractures** may occur. In these situations a child falls on an outstretched arm and immediately experiences pain. The arm may seem okay, but if it remains very tender at a specific point, the child should be taken for X-rays. In these fractures, one side of the bone breaks, but the break does not go all the way through. These should be cared for by an orthopedist, as improper treatment could result in unbalanced growth of the bone, causing the arm to curve. All fractures require immediate orthopedic care.

Chronic elbow pain in childhood is most often the result of overuse. The bones and ligaments of young children lack the strength to endure the repeated stress associated with throwing hard and other sports-related activities. While the number of innings pitched during games is strictly limited in organized baseball, many parents fail to recognize that too many hard pitches in practice can also cause damage. Symptoms of **Little Leaguer's elbow** include pain or swelling along the inner aspect of the elbow and difficulty straightening the arm fully. Although X-rays may be normal, children with these complaints should be made to rest and not be allowed to throw until the symptoms have entirely disappeared. Continuing to throw despite elbow pain most likely will lead to long-term disability.

Older children in throwing sports such as football and baseball may develop **osteochondritis dissecans** of the elbow as a result of repeated stress on the bone from overuse. See discussion under "Knee Pain."

Tennis elbow is a degenerative change at the origin of the muscle that is used to flex the wrist for activities such as backhanding a tennis shot. This muscle (the extensor carpi radialis brevis) is anchored to the arm just below the elbow. Excessive jerking of the muscle with strong contractions causes pain and irritation where it attaches to the bone. This is rarely seen in young children but may occur in adolescents who are overusing the arm. **Golfer's elbow** is a similar injury occurring on the inside of the elbow with a different group of muscles. As with all such overuse injuries, these problems are best treated with rest and modification of the activity to prevent further injury.

Juvenile arthritis infrequently begins in the elbow joint without findings of pain, swelling, or limitation of motion elsewhere. However, any child who exhibits swelling of the elbow and difficulty straightening the arm fully should be carefully evaluated for other explanations. Children with arthritis beginning in the elbow may be labeled as having pauciarticular-onset arthritis, but such children most often go on to have more widespread joint disease over time (see Chapter 5).

Shoulder Pain

Fractures in the area of the shoulder are usually the obvious result of direct trauma and always require orthopedic intervention. The most common chronic conditions producing pain in the shoulder are overuse injuries associated with sports, though any child with recurrent problems should be evaluated for the presence of underlying conditions.

The great range of movement possible at the shoulder is due to the fact that unlike the hip, the shoulder is not limited by a deep bone socket. As a result, the shoulder is much more dependent on strong ligaments to maintain proper alignment. Young people with relatively loose ligaments are therefore uniquely susceptible to recurrent shoulder injury and dislocation, especially if they are involved in athletics. Any child with recurrent shoulder dislocations without obvious explanation should be evaluated for ligamentous laxity and associated conditions (see Chapter 16).

Little Leaguer's shoulder is an inflammation of the growth plate in the shoulder. It results in pain when the shoulder is pressed and, in more severe cases, weakness. Advanced cases are easily diagnosed on X-ray, but any child experiencing pain should be restricted from further throwing and other stressful shoulder activities until the pain has resolved.

Rotator cuff injuries are typically the result of irritation of the muscles in the rotator cuff because they are being compressed between the upper bone of the arm (humerus) and the scapula (the bone that attaches the arm to the body; see Fig. 3-11). This compression is thought to result from imbalances in the strength of the muscles and ligaments that normally keep the bones properly aligned. Most often children report pain with throwing and other overhand activities. Allowed to rest and rehabilitate appropriately, most children can resume full activity. X-rays are rarely helpful in diagnosing this condition; MRI may be warranted if the problems persist. Surgical intervention is infrequently necessary unless the rotator cuff has been torn by continued overuse.

Hand, Wrist, and Finger Pain

Finger injuries are extremely common in children of all ages. Obvious fractures are easily recognized and quickly diagnosed by appropriate X-ray examination.

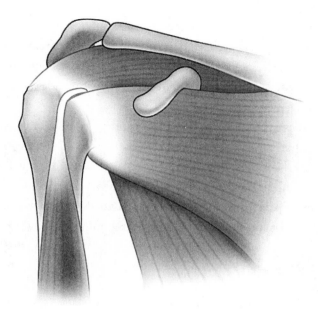

FIG 3-11 *The muscles of the shoulder and the rotator cuff. Injuries often result from the muscles enlarging with athletic activity to the point where they are irritated as they pass between the bones.*

Children with persistent finger injuries require careful evaluation. Children with blunt trauma to the ends of the fingers may suffer damage to the tendons, resulting in **mallet finger** (the tip of the finger is pointed down and cannot be brought up) or **boutonniere deformity** (the tip of the finger is pulled up [see Fig. 13.2]). Whenever a child suffers an injury to the end of the finger, parents should check that the child can move all of the individual parts of the finger appropriately. If a tendon is ruptured, the injury should be corrected surgically. Boutonniere deformity may also be the result of arthritis.

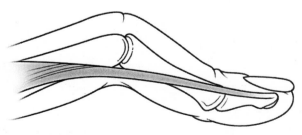

FIG 3-12 *Boutonniere deformity, resulting from tendon slippage.*

Young children with swollen fingers or toes without explanation are often thought to have banged or stubbed them. But if the pain or swelling persists, the child should be carefully examined for evidence of arthritis. Persistent swollen fingers (**dactylitis**, or "sausage digit") may be the first manifestation of serious arthritis (see Chapter 7).

Wrist injuries are common among older children engaged in vigorous sports activity. Most fractures are easily diagnosed with X-rays. One exception is fractures of the scaphoid bone, located at the center of the wrist. Fractures usually occur when a child falls hard on the outstretched hand. Although the child may complain of pain in the wrist, there is often no obvious problem. However, the pain will persist and the wrist will be tender if it is moved in the direction of the thumb or pressure is applied to the space at the base of the thumb (see Fig. 3-13). Fractures of the scaphoid often are not seen on regular X-rays unless special views are taken.

Another fracture that may not be immediately recognized is the **boxer's fracture**, which occurs at the first knuckle of the little finger (end of the fifth metacarpal). This fracture frequently occurs when the child strikes something hard, such as a wall or a locker. There is marked pain over the base of the finger. This fracture should be identified and properly treated, as failure to correct the injury may result in significant deformity.

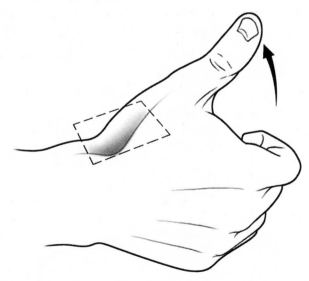

FIG 3-13 *Pain in the base of the thumb is an important finding suggesting a fracture of the scaphoid bone in the wrist.*

Tendon irritation, sprains, and strains are uncommon in children under the age of ten except as the result of trauma. In older children, overuse injuries are common, especially with tennis and gymnastics. Children experiencing wrist pain in association with sports activities should be allowed to rest and recuperate to avoid worsening the inflammation.

Several forms of arthritis commonly begin in the wrist. The key to recognizing arthritis early lies in a careful examination. Most children with arthritis have several joints involved, whereas children with a chronic injury usually have only one involved joint.

Certain genetic conditions may initially present with complaints of hand and wrist pain without obvious explanation. Metabolic storage diseases may cause a buildup of abnormal materials that first cause pain in the hands because the wrist is a narrow space where nerves can be compressed. Although Fabry disease and mucopolysaccharidosis type I are very rare conditions, children with these diseases are often found to have been complaining of unexplained hand pain for years before the other manifestations of the diseases became obvious.

A NOTE ABOUT SPORTS AND PAIN IN CHILDREN

Sports injuries are the most common causes of muscle, bone, and joint pains in childhood. Some of these, particularly overuse injuries, are described in the preceding sections. Often these are minor injuries that resolve over a few hours or days at most. However, pain that is severe or persists requires medical attention. Also, any child who is repeatedly injured or in pain every time he or she participates needs to be evaluated to find out why.

You may have heard the saying "No pain, no gain." While it is true that a certain amount of muscle pain with activity may be associated with building stronger muscles, *bone or joint pain is never associated with gain.* Continued activity on bones or joints that hurt is causing injury and may be causing permanent damage, despite what athletic coaches or trainers may say. Parents, coaches, and children all need to recognize that while athletic activity is clearly beneficial, an overemphasis on achievement may put children at risk for chronic injuries that will prevent them from achieving their athletic goals in the short term and perhaps even persist throughout adulthood.

4

The Child Who Hurts All Over

Children who complain of constant pain are a source of great concern for both parents and physicians. While there are many possible explanations, these symptoms may be the first indication of rheumatic or other serious diseases. Parents who are concerned should schedule a full physical examination, making sure the staff knows this is not a routine physical. Your child is far more likely to get the care he or she needs if your physician knows why you are coming and is thinking about the problem in advance.

One of the greatest difficulties for families and physicians is that some children with widespread complaints do not look ill. Routine physical examination of the heart, lungs, and abdomen will not reveal what is causing the child so much distress, for these will not provide evidence of muscle pain, weakness, or tender joints. Some conditions such as celiac disease or mild variants of the mucopolysaccharidoses and other genetic diseases will be diagnosed only if they are tested for; routine testing will not reveal them. You may need to insist on blood tests, X-rays, or a specialist referral.

I have developed my own standardized list of tests to evaluate children who simply are not doing well (see box). However, it is not practical to recommend that a physician do all of these tests on every child who does not feel well and complains of pain.

Tests for the Evaluation of Children Who Are Just Not Doing Well

PPD (skin test for tuberculosis)
Complete blood count (CBC)
Erythrocyte sedimentation rate (ESR)
T3, T4, TSH, antithyroid antibodies, antithyroid peroxidase (thyroid function studies)
IgA tissue transglutaminase (antiendomysial antibodies, associated with celiac disease)
Creatine kinase (CK) and aldolase (muscle enzymes)
Complete chemistry panel (a broad panel of general tests, including liver and kidney function)
Glucose, calcium, albumin, and total protein
Electrolytes including sodium, potassium, carbon dioxide, and chloride
Kidney tests including blood urea nitrogen (BUN) and creatinine

---

Liver tests including alkaline phosphatase (ALP), alanine amino transferase (ALT, also
called SGPT), aspartate amino transferase (AST, also called SGOT), lactic acid
dehydrogenase (LDH), and bilirubin
Urinanalysis (UA)
Serologic markers including antinuclear antibody (ANA), rheumatoid factor (RF), and
Lyme titer
Amylase and lipase (for children with abdominal pain, dry eyes, or dry mouth)
Total immunoglobulin levels including IgG, IgA, IgM (for children with frequent
infections)
Clotting studies prothrombin time (PT) and partial thromboplastin time (PTT) (for
children with bruising, bleeding, heavy menstrual periods, or chest pain)
HLA B27 (for children with joint pain)
Urine for glycosaminoglycans
Genetic tests (for children with a relevant family history)

The majority of children with a significant illness of the musculoskeletal
system have specific findings on physical examination or abnormalities on at
least some of these laboratory tests. Sometimes the abnormalities will seem only
minor, but they must be viewed as part of a pattern. However, even if the values
on these laboratory tests are normal, that is not always enough to rule out a
significant medical condition; some children with spondyloarthropathies or
other conditions do not have any laboratory abnormalities. Nonetheless, these
children can be easily diagnosed by careful physical examination. Sometimes
children have vague complaints during the earliest stages of a disease, even before
obvious abnormalities occur. It may not be possible to make a definite diagnosis
in these children at this time, but your physician should take your concerns
seriously and follow up rather than simply tell you nothing is wrong.

LABORATORY FINDINGS

As previously noted, normal test results do not necessarily mean the absence of
disease. Many children with chronic diseases begin to lose their energy and feel
unwell long before their routine laboratory results become abnormal. It is important to make sure that all of the appropriate tests have been done. Also, remember that things change over time. Tests that were normal on a first visit may not
be normal four or six months later. In the search for an explanation for a chronically ill child, it is important to reevaluate everything periodically. Often the

earliest abnormalities include a mild elevation of the ESR, a mild anemia, or mild hypoalbuminemia (see Chapter 22). Each of these findings is nonspecific, but an increasing number or gradual worsening of these nonspecific findings should alert the physician.

Many children with normal laboratory testing but continued complaints are labeled as having fibromyalgia or a similar condition. However, it is important to be sure that other significant illnesses have been excluded. Extra steps should be taken if the child has any abnormal laboratory findings, including a positive test for antinuclear antibody (ANA), elevated ESR, or anemia. Even without such abnormalities, consideration must be given to the rarer genetic conditions. Evaluation of such children may include a bone scan and a gallium scan, which may reveal the presence of infections, tumors, or other causes of inflammation. PET scans are now becoming more readily available, and these are very effective in finding areas of increased cell turnover, which could be tumors or infections. Tests such as MRI or ultrasound may be helpful in further evaluating an area that has been identified as abnormal, but the bone scan and gallium scan have the advantage of evaluating the entire body in order to determine where more precise evaluation may be helpful (see Chapter 22). Urine testing for glycosaminoglycans is a useful screen for mild variants of the mucopolysaccharidoses. Blood tests are available for Fabry disease.

WHEN NOTHING IS FOUND

Families and physicians often become frustrated when, despite an entirely normal diagnostic evaluation, a child continues to complain of feeling unwell and is unable to continue his or her normal daily activities. Often the relationship between the family and the physician becomes adversarial: the family knows there is something wrong with the child, but the physician knows he or she cannot find anything wrong. *It is vital for everyone involved to recognize that they are on the same side.*

Often in this situation physicians will recommend a psychological evaluation. Parents often interpret this as a suggestion that they or their child are crazy or that the child must be faking the symptoms. Both physician and family must realize that while psychological illness may cause chronic complaints of pain, chronic pain may also cause psychological illness. However, referral of the child to a psychologist should not stop the ongoing medical evaluation of the child. Looking in only one direction at a time may not be in the child's best interest.

The family must have complete confidence in the physician. If for any reason the family does not, a second opinion should be sought. Every reasonable physician has the child's best interest at heart. If another physician has a useful suggestion, everyone benefits. If the relationship between the physician and family has foundered and the family can establish a better relationship with a new physician, again everyone is better off. Sometimes a specialist will be able to diagnose and treat a number of unusual conditions that other physicians might not recognize.

PART II

THE RHEUMATIC DISEASES AND RELATED CONDITIONS

5

Juvenile Arthritis

Arthritis is defined as pain, swelling, or limitation of motion in a joint. According to the criteria of the American College of Rheumatology, juvenile rheumatoid arthritis (JRA) is the proper diagnosis for any child with the onset of arthritis before sixteen years of age if the arthritis lasts at least six weeks in more than one joint or three months in a single joint, without other explanation.

Based on this definition, every child with chronic arthritis has JRA. However, it is very clear that not every child with arthritis has the same condition. A five-year-old girl with a swollen knee and inflamed eyes does not have the same disease as a teenage boy with a swollen knee and ankle pain. They have different prognoses (probable outcomes in the future), different responses to medication (the best medicine for the little girl is unlikely to be the best medicine for the boy), and most likely different causes for their disease. Rheumatologists recognize more than fifty causes of chronic arthritis in adults, only one of which is rheumatoid arthritis, and there are probably just as many different causes of arthritis in childhood. However, we haven't yet worked out a formal system that differentiates among them, which leads to a lot of confusion and misinformation.

Because most children with arthritis do not have a disease that is in any way related to the rheumatoid arthritis seen in adults, I prefer to use the term **juvenile arthritis (JA)** to refer to idiopathic inflammation of the joints in a child. (*Idiopathic* simply means "unexplained," as opposed to inflammation caused by an infection or other obvious cause; some people prefer the term **juvenile idiopathic arthritis**, or JIA.) I use this term as *JRA* was originally used, that is, to refer to *all* children with unexplained arthritis beginning before the age of sixteen. But it's important to reiterate that JA does not refer to a single disease with a single cause. In fact, JA is not a disease at all; it is a group of signs and symptoms with many different causes and outcomes. Thus, to say that a child has juvenile arthritis is no more meaningful than to say that a child has a broken bone. Just as with the broken bone much depends on which bone is affected and how badly it is broken, in JA much depends on the type of JA and how severe it is.

In our efforts to distinguish the different types of JA, a number of subgroups have been proposed. None of these is truly definitive, and there may well be several distinct diseases within each of the subgroups. In what follows I indicate the generally accepted subgroups in each section, but I also make distinctions based on my personal experience. For our knowledge to advance, however, we will need to identify and investigate these subgroups and refine our divisions further, so that we may identify treatments that are more likely to be effective for a particular child.

PAUCIARTICULAR-ONSET JUVENILE ARTHRITIS

The only divisions currently recognized among JA patients involve how the disease first appears. Children with **pauciarticular onset** have four or fewer joints involved during the first six months, while those with **polyarticular onset** have five or more joints involved during the first six months. The third category is **systemic onset**, which involves daily spiking fevers and rash; the number of joints does not matter.

To base the distinction between pauciarticular-onset and polyarticular-onset JA only on the basis of the number of joints involved six months after onset may seem both confusing and of limited utility. After all, it's hard to tell exactly when someone's arthritis began, and the drawing of the line at five joints seems a bit arbitrary. However, the classification persists because it is generally useful. Children who have arthritis of the hands and feet, whether or not the large joints are affected, usually have more joints involved (because of the number of joints in those areas) and thus fall into the category of polyarticular onset. These children have a different prognosis (and probably a different disease) than children with only large joint involvement, who tend to fall into the category of pauciarticular onset because there are not that many large joints in the body. The proper classification should be onset with only large joints versus onset with small joints involved, with or without large joints.

Pauciarticular-onset arthritis may take a variety of different forms, but it is most often a disease of young girls and some boys that starts between one and seven years of age. (Older children with disease only in large joints often have one of the spondyloarthropathies. This is a completely different group of diseases with different outcomes and different best therapies. These are discussed separately in Chapter 7.) In the most typical cases of pauciarticular disease, the child has one swollen knee. Frequently, there is no history of pain and the parents have been unaware of the problem until a friend or relative pointed out the swollen joint. When asked, the parents cannot tell you when the problem began. There may be awareness that the child walks funny when he or she first gets up, but because the limp disappears after a little while, the parents think it's not significant. Some physicians have referred to this as "painless JRA" because the child does not complain. However, if you squeeze the joint or attempt to manipulate it through the normal range of motion, it is painful. The child does not complain because he or she does not recognize that this is not the way the knee is supposed to feel.

Children who suddenly develop a painful, swollen knee should not be considered as having pauciarticular JA, as the pain and swelling could be caused by infection (including Lyme disease), reactive arthritis, foreign body synovitis, or injury. On rare occasions a child who has acute pain in conjunction with an infection will be discovered to also have pauciarticular arthritis. The chronic disease frequently can be recognized because of bony overgrowth, which occurs over a long period as the body manufactures extra bone to limit joint movement.

Children who develop sudden pain in the hip also should not be considered as having pauciarticular JA. Although polyarticular-onset arthritis and systemic-onset arthritis may ultimately involve the hip, it is never the first joint involved, and the hip is never involved in pauciarticular arthritis. I have seen cases of toxic synovitis, Lyme disease, osteoid osteoma, fractures, and tumors misdiagnosed as juvenile arthritis starting in the hip. Spondyloarthropathies may start in the hip, but these are most often in children over the age of ten years.

Laboratory findings in children with pauciarticular-onset disease are usually normal or display only mild abnormalities. If a child has significant laboratory abnormalities during the first six months of treatment, the diagnosis of pauciarticular JA should be regarded with suspicion. Children who have a hemoglobin level below 11 gm/dl without explanation, a sedimentation rate greater than 40 mm/hr, immunoglobulin A (IgA) deficiency, the genetic marker HLA B27, or a family history of psoriasis or inflammatory bowel disease likely do not have true pauciarticular-onset disease and are at greater risk for additional arthritis-related problems in the future. By contrast, the prognosis for children with well-defined pauciarticular-onset disease is good.

Complications of Pauciarticular-Onset JA

Two well-known complications of typical pauciarticular-onset disease are limb length discrepancy (one leg grows longer than the other) and eye inflammation. Other possible complications include neck and jaw problems.

Limb length discrepancy in children with pauciarticular arthritis is most often seen if the inflammation is in one knee and is not brought under control quickly. The inflamed knee develops increased blood flow as a result of substances produced by the inflamed synovium (the membrane that lines the joint). This increased blood flow brings more nutrients to the bones around the knee and they will grow more rapidly, causing the leg to be longer on that side.

The best way to detect discrepancies in leg length is by measuring the exact length of the leg, either through a scanogram (a special type of X-ray) or a CAT scan (which is faster and more accurate). Such differences are not always visible just by watching a child walk, because children with arthritis in the knee often develop a flexion contracture, which makes the leg appear shorter. A child may constantly hold the inflamed knee in a bent position because it hurts less, and this plus muscle spasms in the knee may shorten and tighten the tendons around the knee, eventually preventing the knee from moving into a fully straight position. (Flexion contractures may also develop in the arm if the elbow is involved.) Anti-inflammatory medications and physical therapy can prevent this problem.

If a child has developed a leg length discrepancy, a lift in the shoe on the shorter side will correct the child's gait. This can help improve the flexion contracture and help avoid hip damage in later life.

Testing for a Knee Flexion Contracture

Have your child sit on the floor with legs together and outstretched. A normal child can put the back of his or her knee flat on the floor so you cannot even slip a piece of paper underneath it. If you can see a space under the knee or slip your fingers under it, there is a flexion contracture.

Children who continually favor the leg that hurts will eventually develop a weakening (atrophy) of the muscles in that leg. As with flexion contracture, physical therapy can help prevent this problem.

An arthritis-affected knee can appear larger than a normal knee because of the muscle atrophy or bony overgrowth, but it can also be larger because of fluid in the joint.

Eye involvement is the other significant complication of pauciarticular JA. Although we do not fully understand why the eye is affected, the presence of a positive ANA is strongly correlated with the risk of eye disease (see Chapter 6). The eye disease, called uveitis or iridocyclitis, takes the form of inflammation of cells in the anterior chamber of the eye. The inflammation can lead to damage to the iris with scarring and irregularity of the pupil. These scars are called synechiae (see Fig. 5-1). Because the eye disease is usually painless and may go unnoticed for a long period, it is recommended that an ophthalmologist screen ANA-positive children every three months. Although the risk of eye involvement is lower in ANA-negative children and in children with polyarticular-onset disease, it may still occur, and ANA-negative children should be screened every six months. Note that it is rare for children with pauciarticular arthritis to develop new eye disease after ten years of age.

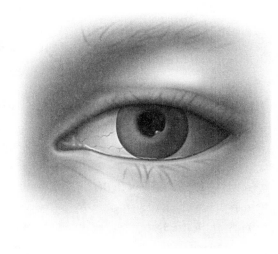

FIG 5-1 *Synechia in the eye of a child with uveitis.*

On occasion I see children who were diagnosed with pauciarticular-onset disease many years before who now have stiff necks. It is well recognized that children with polyarticular-onset disease may develop cervical fusion over time, causing the stiff neck. Sometimes there is no real complaint from the child, and the finding is noted only on X-rays. It is unclear whether cervical fusion is a complication of true pauciarticular-onset arthritis or whether these are children whose disease should have been characterized as polyarticular initially.

Some children with pauciarticular-onset arthritis eventually develop problems with the temporomandibular joint, which allows the jaw to open and close. It can present as difficulty opening the mouth widely, difficulty chewing, or chronic headaches on one side of the head. Often this occurs in children who are also found to have neck pain. How these two findings are interrelated and their relationship to true pauciarticular-onset arthritis is unclear. Temporomandibular joint involvement also occurs in some children with spondyloarthropathies.

Treatment for Pauciarticular-Onset Arthritis

Treatment for pauciarticular-onset arthritis usually consists of nonsteroidal anti-inflammatory drugs (NSAIDs). These drugs are discussed in detail in Chapter 20. I often use diclofenac for children with pauciarticular-onset disease that does not respond adequately to other NSAIDs. Naproxen, celecoxib, nabumetone, and diclofenac have the advantage of being given less frequently than ibuprofen.

For children who have true pauciarticular arthritis, it is rare for additional medications to be necessary. Occasionally, there are children who have persistent swelling of one or two joints despite an adequate trial of NSAIDs. This is the point at which it is reasonable to consider injection of corticosteroids directly into the joint (intra-articular injection). These rarely have side effects and often provide rapid and dramatic relief for months. Most children can be talked through injection of one joint without undue distress, but anesthesia may be necessary if more than one joint must be injected. If more than two joints are persistently inflamed, this suggests that the child has polyarticular disease, not pauciarticular JA, and systemic medication is more likely to give a better long-term response than multiple injections.

Most pediatric rheumatologists believe that appropriate use of intra-articular corticosteroids will decrease the frequency of leg length discrepancy by bringing resistant inflammation under control more rapidly. Intra-articular corticosteroids in conjunction with physical therapy and night splints or serial casting often make it easier to correct flexion contractures. Night splints are casts cut lengthwise so they can be put on at night and taken off in the morning, holding the leg (or arm) straight while the child sleeps. With serial casting, the muscles are relaxed and the leg is placed in a cast for twenty-four to forty-eight hours. When the cast is cut off, it is often possible to extend the leg a little further. This can be repeated several times.

In children who reach the age of ten with a significant persisting leg length discrepancy, an orthopedic appointment should be scheduled. With data from CAT scans or X-rays, orthopedists can predict the amount of future bone growth. In general, they will not intervene unless they expect a leg length difference of more than one inch. In that case, minor surgery is done to place a staple in the growth plate (distal epiphysis) of the leg that is too long, signaling that bone to stop growing while the shorter one continues to grow.

There are two other situations in which surgery is considered for children with pauciarticular-onset arthritis. If a very severe flexion contracture has developed and it cannot be corrected with physical therapy and intra-articular corticosteroids, the orthopedist may consider doing tendon releases. In addition, there are exceptional cases of children with chronic active synovitis unresponsive to multiple medications or intra-articular corticosteroids. These children probably do not have true pauciarticular-onset arthritis. It may be necessary for the surgeon to explore the joint to determine what is going on, remove some of the excess tissue (synovectomy), and obtain appropriate tissue for examination by the pathologist to exclude other diseases such as plant thorn synovitis (see Chapter 3).

Prognosis for Children with Pauciarticular-Onset JA

The prognosis for the typical child with true pauciarticular arthritis is very good. Most children respond as expected to therapy and are well within a few months. My normal standard is to treat a child until there has been no evidence of active disease for six months. This often means nine months to a year of treatment. At that point, I will discontinue the NSAIDs and watch carefully. Most children (about 80 percent) will remain well without medication. In a few children, the disease will flare up shortly after stopping medication, and a few more children will develop new episodes of arthritis over the next few years. The explanation for this is unclear.

When pauciarticular-onset arthritis flares up in a child, he or she should be carefully reinvestigated to exclude other problems. Children may develop Lyme disease, bone infections, or other problems that at first look like a recurrence of the JA. If other problems have been excluded but the child does not respond quickly to reintroducing NSAIDs, he or she probably did not have true pauciarticular-onset arthritis.

The majority of children with true pauciarticular-onset disease will be able to carry out fully functional lives in every way. The prognosis for children with significant eye disease will depend on their ultimate visual status; this is best discussed with the treating ophthalmologist (see Chapter 6).

POLYARTICULAR-ONSET JUVENILE ARTHRITIS

Polyarticular-onset disease is defined as arthritis involving five or more joints during the first six months of disease, without other explanation. In my opinion, any involvement of small joints indicates polyarticular-type disease even if initially there are fewer than five joints involved. Polyarticular-onset disease may occur in any age group but is found more often in girls than in boys. There are two major peaks in the age at onset of disease: in young children between eighteen months and eight years of age and in older children and teenagers after eleven years of age. Some children start with only one or two arthritic joints, with the arthritis slowly spreading to other joints, while other children rapidly develop arthritis of multiple joints.

Most pediatric rheumatologists make distinctions based on the presence or absence of rheumatoid factor (RF) in the blood (it is normally absent). These children may also be subcategorized according to whether the disease is symmetric (both elbows or both knees, etc.) or asymmetric (only one elbow or one knee, along with other joints). Children with tendon insertion inflammation (enthesitis), a family history of psoriasis, a family history of inflammatory bowel disease, or the presence of HLA B27 are included in this group by some physicians but are excluded by others. I exclude children with these findings because I believe most of them have spondyloarthropathies that behave differently (see Chapter 7). Even when all the children with these findings are excluded, the remaining children are a diverse group and most likely have one of several different diseases.

Laboratory findings in children with polyarticular-onset arthritis are highly variable. Some have entirely normal laboratory tests, while others have elevated ESR and low hemoglobin. A small percentage of children with polyarticular-onset are RF-positive and should be considered as having an early onset of adult-type rheumatoid arthritis. However, RF may be found in a number of other conditions (see Chapter 22) and should not be relied on to establish this diagnosis. A positive test for rheumatoid factor in a child less than ten years of age is far more likely a false positive result or an indication of another illness than a sign of early-onset RF-positive polyarticular arthritis. The test for ANA may also be positive in children with polyarticular-onset disease. Although their risk of eye disease is lower than that of ANA-positive children with pauciarticular-onset disease, ANA-positive children with polyarticular disease also have an increased risk of uveitis and should have an examination by an ophthalmologist every three months.

Several diseases need to be distinguished from polyarticular-onset arthritis. Children with rheumatic diseases such as systemic lupus erythematosus

(Chapter 9), dermatomyositis (Chapter 14), polyarteritis nodosa (inflammation of the arteries), sarcoidosis (a rheumatic disease that may cause elevated calcium levels), and mixed connective tissue disease (Chapter 10) often have polyarticular arthritis in addition to their other symptoms. There are a variety of less common diseases that also may begin with polyarticular arthritis and should be excluded by history, physical, and laboratory evaluation. Children with chronic pains in their hands or feet without obvious synovitis should be evaluated for the possibility of other conditions such as Fabry disease or mucopolysaccharidosis.

The disease most often confused with polyarticular-onset JA is **reactive arthritis** (also called **infection-associated arthritis**). Reactive arthritis often begins with the rapid onset of disease involving the large and small joints (see Chapter 7). The key to suspecting this diagnosis is the occurrence of an infection around ten to fourteen days before the onset of arthritis. Children who rapidly develop polyarticular arthritis should be evaluated carefully for evidence of either a recent infection or an infection that is still present and may need to be treated. Parvovirus B19 infection and Lyme disease are just two examples of many infections that may cause an acute reactive arthritis with an elevated sedimentation rate and an ill-appearing child. Reactive arthritis typically resolves over a period of a few weeks to several months, but in some cases it appears that an infection that is known to cause reactive arthritis initiates chronic polyarticular arthritis in a susceptible individual (see Chapter 7).

Children with early onset of polyarticular disease often seem to improve initially but then worsen in a series of episodes over a period of years, progressively developing more joint involvement. It is usually possible to bring their arthritis under reasonable control with medications, but it is unlikely that their arthritis will ever be completely gone.

Children with early onset of polyarticular-onset disease who have continuing disease activity should be treated relatively aggressively. Often the parents and children become tired of all the medicines and doctor appointments. However, the outcome is generally much better for children who are consistently treated than for those who just take the pills when they are uncomfortable. With medications such as etanercept and adalimumab, we can provide sustained relief of symptoms and slow or prevent joint damage. Children with chronic disease should be on these medications to prevent long-term disability.

Children with the later onset of polyarticular disease are highly varied in their outcomes. Some seem to have arthritis that resolves without explanation, while others with no apparent risk factors progressively develop more severe joint involvement. Therapy with etanercept or adalimumab should be considered for any child who is not obtaining nearly complete symptomatic relief from NSAIDs. In addition, any child with evidence of erosions or other indications of long-term joint damage should be on methotrexate, etanercept, or adalimumab.

Complications of Polyarticular-Onset JA

The complications of polyarticular-onset juvenile arthritis are primarily those of the arthritis itself. Pain, swelling, and limitation of motion may result in weakness, bone loss (osteoporosis), and difficulty in activities of daily living. This type of arthritis may spread to involve the hip in some children, and hip replacement surgery is sometimes necessary to maintain function (see "Treatment of Polyarticular-Onset JA," below). Involvement of the wrists and fingers may also limit function. Cervical spine fusion and foot deformities are additional complications that are seen in some children with chronic active disease. Fortunately, the majority of children experience substantial relief when aggressively treated, and the risk of severe joint damage has diminished substantially with the increased utilization of etanercept and adalimumab.

The key to minimizing complications in children with polyarticular disease is early and aggressive medical intervention. Once it is recognized that a child has progressive polyarticular disease, every effort must be made to suppress the inflammation. The vast majority of children who receive proper treatment do very well.

Treatment of Polyarticular-Onset JA

Medical therapy for severe arthritis has progressed dramatically in the last twenty years. The potential side effects and appropriate monitoring for each of the medications are discussed in detail in Chapter 20. A few children with mild polyarticular-onset arthritis will respond well to NSAIDs; most of these need the stronger NSAIDs (diclofenac is often my first choice), but some find nabumetone, naproxen, or ibuprofen adequate. For children with more severe disease, sulfasalazine is often an effective second-line agent. If further medication is necessary, the standard answer is to proceed to methotrexate. However, many families and physicians prefer to use a tumor necrosis factor (TNF) inhibitor (etanercept, adalimumab, or infliximab) early in the disease course. The TNF inhibitors are given by injection and often produce a dramatic, rapid, and sustained improvement. For children who do not respond to TNF inhibitors, other drugs are available that block T cell signaling (abatacept), interleukin-1 (anakinra and others), or interleukin-6 (tocilizumab and others). There is extensive experience with the long-term safety and efficacy of the TNF inhibitors as well as anakinra. The other agents are newer and still undergoing evaluation. Fortunately, few children fail to respond to the TNF inhibitors.

It is rare for these drugs to fail in children with polyarticular disease. When they do, it becomes a matter of careful testing to determine what will help. Cyclosporine is effective for some children, azathioprine for others. A few centers still use intravenous immunoglobulin G (IgG), but it has few lasting effects and most have discontinued its use for polyarticular-onset arthritis. For the few children who fail to respond to routine therapy there are several newer agents, including rituximab. A large number of agents are in the late stages of clinical evaluation and may become available soon.

Corticosteroid-containing drugs such as prednisone will make a child feel better rapidly, but prolonged use is frequently associated with major side effects such as impaired growth, obesity, and avascular necrosis of bone (death of bone tissue). I reserve corticosteroids primarily for children who cannot even get out of bed to go to school in the morning, but I nearly always begin a second-line agent shortly afterward, with the intent of stopping the steroids as quickly as possible.

I occasionally see children with arthritis who are taking painkillers. Excessive use of codeine and its derivatives or similar drugs is often associated with abnormal behavior and in some cases can lead to addiction, so I do not use them. More importantly, I believe it is better to fix the problem than simply to mask the pain. For most children with arthritis, acetaminophen is an appropriate and adequate addition to help control pain. However, I do have a few patients who require tramadol or propoxyphene on occasion.

Parents may be concerned by the prospect of their children taking medications for a long time. Once joint damage has occurred, it cannot be reversed, and the child will suffer with the consequences for the rest of his or her life. The medications are prescribed to avoid the damage occurring in the first place. For this reason I strongly counsel parents to listen when a physician prescribes aggressive therapy.

Surgical therapy for children with polyarticular-onset arthritis is primarily limited to joint replacement surgery. Before I discuss these, however, I want to reiterate that appropriate use of TNF inhibitors and other drugs can make it much less likely that a child will have to undergo surgery.

Children with severe involvement of the shoulder may benefit from replacement of the head of the shoulder (glenoid). This is the one joint replacement surgery in the upper extremity that is useful. Upper extremity joint replacement below the shoulder is generally unsatisfactory. However, children with fused elbows may benefit from elbow replacement surgery to restore some movement, as significant loss of range of motion in both elbows makes it very difficult to carry out daily activities such as eating and dressing.

Children with severe involvement of the wrist or fingers may benefit from fusion of particularly troublesome joints. Replacement of finger joints is not generally helpful. When there is significant subluxation (downward slipping) of the wrist, surgery to fuse the wrist in a functional position is often helpful. In addition, it is sometimes necessary to remove the tip of the bone at the end of the forearm (distal ulna) if it is causing damage to the tendons that extend the fingers as the tendons pass over the bone.

Joint replacement surgery for the lower extremities is much more effective. If a child is losing the ability to walk because of hip pain, it is important to replace the hip as soon as possible. Waiting does not make sense, for as soon as the disease limits the amount of walking the child can do, strength and range of motion are lost. This makes recovery after surgery much more difficult and complete functional recovery much less likely (see Chapter 23).

Physical and occupational therapy play an important role in children with polyarticular-onset disease, helping maintain children's strength, endurance, and range of motion. Sometimes parents may feel that their children do all sorts of physical and occupational (not to mention medical) therapy and never seem to get better. It is important to realize that children with arthritis who are left untreated steadily get worse. Sometimes in the face of very active disease, therapy succeeds in slowing down the progression of the problem until new medications take effect or the disease itself remits somewhat. These children are much better off because of their therapy, even though they may have gotten worse while being treated.

Splinting is an important part of physical and occupational therapy. Children with pain often hold their joints in the position of maximum comfort. This is not the position of maximum function. See the discussion of splinting in "Treatment for Pauciarticular-Onset Arthritis," above. Children often protest vociferously about splinting, because it is not comfortable and sometimes the joint feels a little stiffer immediately after taking off the splint. It is essential to remember, however, that splinting improves function.

Prognosis for Children with Polyarticular-Onset JA

The long-term prognosis for children with polyarticular-onset disease is highly variable, with a long list of possible complications. Remember, however, that most of the long-term complications can be prevented by early use of TNF inhibitors and additional agents if necessary. If significant joint damage has occurred prior to or despite proper therapy, surgical intervention may be helpful.

SYSTEMIC-ONSET JUVENILE ARTHRITIS

Systemic-onset juvenile arthritis refers to the onset of arthritis with fever and a characteristic rash. Systemic-onset juvenile arthritis has no relationship to adult-onset rheumatoid arthritis and most likely no relationship to the other forms of juvenile arthritis, either. It is best considered an entirely separate disease.

Although all children with systemic-onset arthritis share key characteristics, the outcome of systemic-onset disease is so varied that it is difficult to believe it is in fact a single disease. There are several key points when making the diagnosis of systemic-onset arthritis. First, the fever must fall back to normal at least once each day. Second, the rash should have the characteristic salmon pink appearance; it should never look like a bruise. It is occasionally itchy. Occasionally, there are children who develop fever and rash before the arthritis becomes evident. These children should always be followed carefully for the possibility of another diagnosis, especially an infection.

Pauciarticular- and polyarticular-onset arthritis affect girls more frequently than boys. In systemic-onset arthritis, the sex ratio is equal. In pauciarticular- and polyarticular-onset disease, a positive ANA test is common and eye disease is frequent. Both ANA and eye disease are rare in systemic-onset juvenile arthritis. Rheumatoid factor should not be present in children with systemic-onset arthritis. If RF is found in a child being investigated for systemic-onset disease, it is more likely that the cause of the symptoms is an infection.

The typical child with systemic-onset arthritis has recurring fevers and a rising ESR, white blood cell (WBC) count, and platelet count, but falling hemoglobin. Often the child looks extremely ill. Most often the child is thought to have an infection, and the possibility of systemic-onset arthritis is considered only when there has been no response to antibiotics.

The first real indication that the diagnosis is systemic-onset arthritis may be the appearance of the characteristic rash. Children with recurrent fevers that fall back to normal should be examined carefully. If the rash is not obvious, parents and physicians should look for it under the arms and around the waist. The rash is often visible only when the child is hot (such as after a bath or after playing sports). Textbooks describe the Koebner phenomenon, in which if you gently scratch the skin, red spots appear around the area that you touched, but in clinical practice this test is rarely positive. Arthritis may be present even at the earliest stages of the disease. Often it is present but has been overlooked. But sometimes it is absent until later in the course of the disease.

A key finding in establishing the diagnosis of systemic-onset arthritis is the child's dramatic improvement during the period when the fever is gone each day. Children with reactive arthritis, infections, or leukemia may be misdiagnosed as having systemic-onset disease; however, these diseases rarely have periods without fever during which the child looks nearly normal, and they are usually associated with a decreased platelet count, whereas systemic-onset arthritis is characteristically associated with a significant elevation of the platelet count.

Until the diagnosis of systemic-onset arthritis is clear, it is far better to continue to look for infections and treat with antibiotics if necessary. It is also far better to have done a bone marrow aspiration to exclude the possibility of leukemia than to delay that diagnosis, thinking the child has systemic-onset arthritis. Children sent to me for possible systemic-onset arthritis have had cancers, infections, polyarteritis nodosa, Kawasaki's disease, inflammatory bowel disease, and many other illnesses.

In addition to the high WBC count, high platelet count, high ESR, and low hemoglobin, laboratory evaluation of the child with systemic-onset arthritis may show mild elevation of the liver enzymes (AST/ALT; see Chapter 22). Significant elevation of these tests in a child with systemic-onset arthritis is a cause for concern. It may signal the beginning of a severe complication called macrophage activation syndrome (MAS; see below).

Complications of Systemic-Onset JA

The complications of systemic-onset arthritis may take many forms. In addition to the problems of fever, rash, and arthritis, many children will have a small pericardial effusion (fluid around the heart) on an echocardiogram. These are often insignificant, but if they become large they may cause difficulty. An enlarged liver or spleen may be found. An excess of protein in the urine is a major cause for concern, as there is a strong association between systemic-onset arthritis and amyloidosis (deposits of protein in the kidneys or other organs), but this is an uncommon disease in developed countries.

There are reports linking systemic-onset arthritis to heart or heart valve damage, lung involvement including pleural effusions, central nervous system problems such as seizures, and a number of vasculitic complications. Whether these are true complications of systemic-onset arthritis is uncertain, because many times what is reported as an atypical complication of systemic-onset arthritis is really a typical complication of systemic vasculitis with arthritis or another disease in a child mistakenly thought to have systemic-onset arthritis. It is important that children with these symptoms be followed carefully and monitored for the possibility of another diagnosis.

Macrophage activation syndrome (MAS) is the most worrisome acute complication of systemic-onset arthritis. If a child with typical systemic-onset arthritis seems to be responding to therapy but the ESR, platelet count, and WBC count begin to fall rapidly while the liver enzymes are increasing, this should spark great concern. The physician may suspect the elevated liver enzymes are an indication of mild liver irritation caused by the medications, but this may instead be the beginning of MAS. This is especially true if the child appears ill.

Most often the onset of MAS occurs early in the course of systemic-onset arthritis, but it may occur at any time. The typical presentation is in a child with systemic-onset arthritis who rapidly appears ill with fever, abnormal liver enzymes, and liver enlargement. MAS frequently occurs shortly after a change in medication or in conjunction with a viral illness; however, the cause is not always evident. In the early stages of MAS, the tests for fibrin degradation products (FDP), fibrin split products (FSP), D-dimers, or prothrombin time (PT) may be abnormal (see Chapter 22). This will not be the case if the child's systemic-onset arthritis is improving. A definitive diagnosis of MAS requires a bone marrow aspiration to demonstrate the presence of macrophages that are destroying red blood cells and their precursors in the marrow. However, it is rarely necessary to perform this test, as the clinical picture is quite striking.

MAS can be a severe and life-threatening problem because of the clotting abnormalities and liver damage that occur. It is treated with high doses of intravenous corticosteroids and fresh frozen plasma. Some children with MAS have improved with cyclosporine therapy. New research suggests there may be predisposing genetic factors and that under the right circumstances, MAS may occur in any child with the genetic predisposition, even if he or she doesn't have systemic-onset arthritis.

The complications of inadequately treated systemic-onset juvenile arthritis include severe damage to both large and small joints. Hips and knees are frequently affected and may require replacement. The cervical spine is another frequently affected area, and fusion of the vertebrae in the neck may occur. In some children the wrists are also significantly involved.

Many children with systemic-onset arthritis receive corticosteroids to control the fever and rash, and complications such as impairment of growth, obesity, osteoporosis, and avascular necrosis of the hips may occur with long-term use of these drugs. Some children with systemic-onset disease who have never taken steroids also have some impairment of growth and wind up shorter than would be expected.

Treatment of Systemic-Onset JA

The medications used in the treatment of systemic-onset arthritis are essentially the same as those used to treat polyarticular-onset disease. However, there are a number of key differences. Virtually all of the medicines used to treat JA may irritate the liver, but in children with systemic-onset arthritis, the disease itself often causes irritation of the liver. As a result, children with systemic-onset arthritis must be monitored carefully for signs of liver irritation, especially after any change in medication.

Indomethacin is uniquely effective in treating the fever of systemic-onset arthritis and may be effective when other NSAIDs have not been helpful; however, it has a number of side effects. For children who fail to respond adequately to NSAIDs, methotrexate is the traditional next choice. However, recent studies have demonstrated that IL-1 and IL-6 play a major role in the manifestations of systemic-onset arthritis, and anakinra and other drugs that block the IL-1 receptors may be dramatically effective in some children. Tocilizumab, which blocks the IL-6 receptors, is in clinical trials and has been very effective for children with systemic-onset disease, though it does have worrisome side effects and as of this writing is not yet licensed in the United States. Thalidomide may dramatically improve the symptoms of children with systemic-onset arthritis but should only be prescribed by an experienced physician. Additionally, cyclosporine, adalimumab, etanercept, and infliximab have all been used with success in some children. In a few children with severe systemic-onset arthritis the disease can be controlled only with long-term use of corticosteroids, but every alternative should be considered first. There are several other medications as well, such as leflunomide, azathioprine, mycophenolate mofetil, and cyclophosphamide, though none is consistently effective. It is rare for a child not to respond to any of these. The goal is to relieve symptoms and eliminate inflammation with the least possible toxicity. (See Chapter 20 for a discussion of all the medications briefly mentioned here.)

Bone marrow transplantation and other dramatic therapies have been proposed for children with the most severe disease. These treatments eliminate the immune system, and because immune system overactivity is responsible for rheumatic diseases, the treatments can eliminate systemic-onset arthritis as well. However, the immune system is how our bodies fight infection, and elimination of the immune system for even a short period (as is done in bone marrow transplantation) carries a high risk—nearly 20 percent of the children who underwent bone marrow transplantation for systemic-onset arthritis died, and others have relapsed. This is not a miracle cure. It is an experimental procedure that should be reserved for the very worst cases.

Physical and occupational therapy are very important in maintaining strength and range of motion for children with systemic-onset arthritis. Without proper therapy, these children may develop widespread weakness, muscle atrophy, and flexion contractures.

Surgery has little direct role in the treatment of children with systemic-onset arthritis. But once the systemic manifestations have come under control, these children may be left with significant polyarticular arthritis. Reconstructive surgery as discussed for children with polyarticular-onset arthritis is appropriate for children with systemic-onset arthritis. Because many of these children have required extended periods of therapy with corticosteroids, they often have avascular necrosis of bone and require joint replacement surgery (see Chapter 23).

Prognosis for Children with Systemic-Onset JA

The course of systemic-onset arthritis is highly varied. Some children make a complete recovery in a short period of time and never have further problems. Other children have chronic debilitating disease that leaves them with permanent limitations. There are three general groups of children with systemic-onset arthritis, but not all children fit one of these descriptions. The first group consists of children who have an acute onset of fever, rash, and arthritis that responds quickly to treatment with NSAIDs. In many cases the duration of disease is less than three months. Some have argued that these are unusual viral infections mimicking systemic-onset arthritis. An outbreak of what was initially thought to be an epidemic of systemic-onset arthritis in a boarding school was found to be due to parvovirus infection when it was carefully investigated. All of these children recovered. Perhaps all of the children who rapidly recover never really had systemic-onset arthritis. We don't know.

The second group of systemic-onset arthritis patients consists primarily of teenage boys. Although their disease may be significant initially, it most often comes under control with NSAIDs. A few require the addition of a second-line agent, but their primary problems are fever and rash with relatively little arthritis. Many of these teenagers find that they do well except for the recurrence of rash whenever they are very hot from exercise. Some have mild persisting arthritis or limitation in their wrists, but they do not have major arthritic problems.

The third group is a much more problematic set of children who begin with systemic-onset disease early in life. In many of these children, multiple medications can achieve control of the disease before there is significant damage to bones and joints, though some require continuing treatment for years, and a few suffer from chronic destructive arthritis. The key to an improved prognosis for this group is early recognition and aggressive intervention while avoiding chronic high-dose corticosteroid therapy whenever possible.

The long-term prognosis for most children with systemic-onset disease is very good. The systemic symptoms usually disappear over a period of time, and the remaining problems are those of polyarticular arthritis. Only a small percentage of children develop prolonged unresponsive arthritis or life-threatening complications. With the advent of newer therapies and increasing recognition of the importance of intervening early to minimize use of corticosteroids, most children with systemic-onset arthritis will be able to live full and productive lives. To get the best possible outcome, the small group of children with severe resistant disease should be shifted to the care of very experienced specialists as soon as they are recognized.

STATE-OF-THE-ART CARE FOR CHILDREN WITH JUVENILE ARTHRITIS

State-of-the-art care for children with pauciarticular-onset, polyarticular-onset, and systemic-onset juvenile arthritis requires that physicians and families make sure the inflammation is promptly brought under control and not allowed to cause continuing joint damage. In the past physicians believed that children who had evidence of low-grade active disease but seemed to be doing okay should not be treated aggressively. We now know this is wrong, as the earliest damage is to the rapidly growing cartilage, and this kind of damage does not show up on X-rays until years later, when it has become permanent bone damage. Failing to treat properly means continuing bone and joint damage and a continuing risk of further disease flares.

Children whose disease comes under good control within six months of starting therapy will generally do well. Children with any type of juvenile arthritis whose disease is not under good control within six months of starting appropriate therapy are at increased risk of a poor outcome. Appropriate therapy can be difficult to define, but to me it means the right NSAID in the right dosage. It also means monitoring carefully and changing the NSAID if it does not appear to be having the desired effect.

Because there are studies that indicate that NSAIDs may not reach their full effectiveness until they have been taken consistently for three months, some physicians will not consider changing therapy until three months after the first dose. However, we must not allow growing children to have continuing joint damage for any longer than is absolutely necessary. If a child is not beginning to improve within three or four weeks of starting an NSAID, another should be tried.

Any child who is not clearly improving after six months of disease may need to be on a second-line agent. However, before I regard a child as needing a second-line agent, I want to have tried two or three first-line agents. Different children have different responses to these medications, so I want to see the child at least monthly at the beginning, and more frequently if he or she is not making good progress. The best possible care requires careful monitoring by both the parents and physician so that any problems are promptly dealt with and appropriate adjustments are made as needed.

In addition to routine checkups, every child should be carefully reevaluated six months after starting therapy. Is the disease under good control? Are the remaining problems simply weakness, contractures, or bony overgrowth? These require physical therapy and time, not more medicine. However, if there is evidence of active disease with an elevated sedimentation rate, unexplained anemia, morning stiffness, joint swelling, or pain, more aggressive therapy with a second-line agent should be considered. For children with pauciarticular-onset arthritis, this might be the time to consider an intra-articular corticosteroid injection. For children with continuing active polyarticular or systemic-onset JA six months after diagnosis, a second-line agent should be added, if one has not been added already.

Your physician should not be providing anything less than state-of-the-art care for your child. If your child is prescribed medications that were once used for JA treatment but have since been abandoned, including aspirin (which has a role in arthritis treatment but has significant side effects in the dosages needed), injections of gold-containing compounds, or D-penicillamine, you need to question the treatment.

6

Uveitis

Eye Complications of Juvenile Arthritis and Related Conditions

In juvenile arthritis and related conditions, the eyes may be involved even when there is no evidence of active joint disease. Ocular complications may take several forms. Children with pauciarticular-onset, polyarticular-onset, and psoriatic arthritis are all at risk of developing eye inflammation (chronic anterior uveitis). In this condition, inflamed cells accumulate in the eye and the resultant irritation may cause damage to the colored part of the eye (iris), the lens, and other structures (see Fig. 5-1 in Chapter 5). The most worrisome aspect of this inflammation is that often it does not produce pain or redness, and so it may cause serious eye damage before it is detected.

The key to preventing serious eye damage in children with JA is careful screening for the presence of inflammatory cells by an ophthalmologist (a medical eye doctor). This is done with a special instrument called a slit lamp, which is not regularly available in the office of physicians who do not specialize in eye disease. An additional quick and easy test recommended by some ophthalmologists is for parents to shine a flashlight in the child's eyes at bedtime one night each week. If you shine a light in a normal child's eye, you will see the pupil (black center) shrink dramatically. It should shrink in a perfect circle. If one eye does not shrink or the circle is irregular, this might be evidence of eye involvement. Whatever the cause, any child whose pupils do not shrink equally when you shine a light in them should be evaluated by an ophthalmologist. This test may detect the onset of inflammation in the eye occurring between screening tests, but it is not a substitute for the screening tests.

Frequency of Routine Screening Ophthalmologic Examinations for Children with Juvenile Arthritis

Condition	ANA Status	Age at Onset	Length of Time with Disease	Screening Interval
Pauciarticular-onset and polyarticular-onset disease	Positive	Under age 7	Less than 4 years	Every 3 months
			More than 4 years	Every 6 months
			More than 7 years	Yearly
		Over age 7	Less than 4 years	Every 6 months
			More than 4 years	Yearly
	Negative	Under age 7	Less than 4 years	Every 6 months
			More than 4 years	Yearly
		Over age 7		Yearly
Systemic-onset JA				Yearly

Note: These are recommendations for routine screening of children who are not known to have uveitis. If the child has uveitis, the frequency of follow-up should be determined by the ophthalmologist.

Physicians do not understand why some children get eye disease and others do not. There are certain genetic factors that seem to increase the risk. However, many children with these factors do not get eye disease, and some children without these factors do get eye disease. Attempts to understand why having ANA increases the risk have failed.

If you look carefully at the joint of a child with arthritis, the inflammation is centered in the synovium. This is the lining tissue, the normal function of which is to keep the joint clean of debris. Examination of the eyes of children with uveitis has shown that the inflammation is centered in the ciliary body. This is a tissue in the eye that serves to keep the fluid in the eye clean of debris. Since the two tissues serve a similar function, it is easy to understand how the same disease process might involve both. But if it were that simple, we would expect all children with arthritis to develop eye involvement. In fact, less than half ever have any evidence of eye inflammation. Clearly other factors play a role.

If uveitis is present, it should be treated aggressively. The normal first-line therapy is steroid eye drops. Often a short course of this treatment is enough to bring the disease under control. Unfortunately, steroid eye drops can damage the eye, possibly causing cataracts or glaucoma, if used for an extended period. Because of these complications, if it appears that a short course of treatment with steroid eye drops is inadequate, many ophthalmologists will recommend switching children with severe eye disease to immunosuppressive medications taken by mouth. Often methotrexate is the first medication used after corticosteroids have proven inadequate. Adalimumab and infliximab are also used in this situation with good efficacy. It is my personal preference to use adalimumab, as it seems to have a faster onset of action and produce a better and more sustained response. Some children respond best to the use of the combination of methotrexate and adalimumab. Since the adalimumab works faster, I usually add the methotrexate only when it is apparent that adalimumab alone is not enough. It is uncommon for children to require stronger medications; if they do, they should be under the care of experienced specialists in large centers.

Many children with JA are found to have mild uveitis, but if they are treated appropriately they do very well. However, if the uveitis is very severe, very resistant to therapy, or not found until very late, there is a risk of permanent blindness. Uveitis may occur in one or both eyes and may develop at a time where there is no evidence of active arthritis. This is why routine monitoring is so important—to find eye disease that you do not suspect is present, and to allow the doctor to begin therapy before too much damage accumulates. Eye doctor appointments should not be put off because you have not noticed any problem.

While eye involvement is common and some children develop serious eye involvement, since the introduction of more potent medications I have seen complete blindness in children with arthritis in only two situations: when children fail to go for screening examinations as recommended and when parents take their children off medication against the physician's advice because they are concerned the child might suffer side effects.

Eye involvement may also occur in children with spondyloarthropathies. However, these children usually get acute and painful eye disease (see Chapter 7). Because it is painful, it is usually rapidly detected. Frequent monitoring of children older than ten with spondyloarthropathies who do not have symptoms in their eyes is not required. In contrast, young children with psoriatic arthritis are at high risk of inflammatory eye disease and must be monitored just as if they had typical JA.

Eye disease may also be a complication of other rheumatic diseases in childhood, including sarcoidosis, systemic lupus erythematosus, and Sjögren's syndrome. Children with each of these conditions should have their eyes checked by an ophthalmologist routinely. In some cases, they will have symptoms of their eye disease; in other cases the eye disease may occur without the parents or child being aware of it. Some children develop uveitis without evidence of a rheumatic disease. Since this eye disease looks the same as the eye disease in children with JA, it is treated the same way. The list of diseases that may cause uveitis in childhood is quite long; however, the first step in evaluating a child who is found to have uveitis is a careful evaluation to make sure he or she does not have a rheumatic disease.

7

Spondyloarthropathies

Enthesitis-associated Arthritis

The term *spondyloarthropathy* does not refer to a specific disease. Meaning "arthritis involving the back," it describes a pattern of inflammation that may occur in children with a variety of underlying conditions. For many years, children with spondyloarthropathies were considered to have JA, but now these children are described as having enthesitis-associated arthritis. Although enthesitis-associated arthritis is considered a subtype of juvenile arthritis, it is important to recognize that this is a very different disease from, for example, pauciarticular-onset arthritis. Remember, *juvenile arthritis* is being used as an umbrella term encompassing a large number of different conditions. In contrast to other types of arthritis, the spondyloarthropathies have a different pattern of joint involvement, a different prognosis, a different best medication, and a different cause.

The first widely recognized group of children with spondyloarthropathies were teenage boys with swollen knees and low back pain. They stood out because under the old nomenclature they were classified as pauciarticular-onset arthritis, even though typical pauciarticular-onset arthritis occurs in young girls. We now know that teenage boys with swollen knees have spondyloarthropathies. (The condition does occur in girls, but rarely in severe form.) Unlike young girls with pauciarticular-onset arthritis, who usually get better, the boys often have persistent chronic arthritis. The boys rarely are ANA-positive, and if they get eye disease, it is acute and painful, not the silent eye disease seen in younger children. In addition, their disease may start in the hip and is often associated with back pain.

When rheumatologists began to look more carefully at this group of teenage boys, they discovered that they often had inflammation in the tendons around the joint (enthesitis) as well as in the joint. Recognition that these boys were different was hastened by the discovery of HLA B27, a genetic marker that is found in about half of this group but only infrequently in young girls with arthritis. Once this group was recognized, pediatric rheumatologists realized that spondyloarthropathies with pain due to inflammation of the tendon insertions (often without obvious arthritis) are common in childhood.

Spondyloarthropathies typically begin in the early teenage years and are often mistaken for recurrent athletic injuries. Unlike typical pauciarticular-onset arthritis, in which it is uncommon for there to be another affected family member, other family members of children with spondyloarthropathies are frequently found to be symptomatic. The affected relatives have had chronic back or knee problems since they were teenagers that they attribute to injuries or other vague causes; they often are unaware that these are signs of a specific medical condition.

The significant findings in children with spondyloarthropathies often relate to tendon inflammation rather than arthritis. Enthesitis causes pain around the wrists, knees, ankles, or heels. Frequently, physicians are confused because the child is complaining of a lot of pain, but nothing is broken and the joint is not swollen. Careful palpation around the joint will often reveal the painful tendonitis. Sometimes the tendons are very swollen and easily noticed on examination. In other cases the tendonitis is obvious only when the tendons are compressed and the child says it hurts.

Pain around the joint (periarticular pain) is the hallmark of spondyloarthropathies. The key to recognizing that the child is not suffering from recurrent athletic injuries is that multiple tender joints are present (for example, it's not just the left ankle that hurts; the right ankle, heel, low back, and wrist may also be tender when examined). Another common finding is pain at the Achilles tendon insertion on the back of the heel or at the insertion of the plantar fascia on the bottom of the foot (see Fig. 7-1). This can be detected by percussion or deep palpation at either point. Discovering that there are similarly affected family members when taking the family history also may speed recognition of a spondyloarthropathy.

Dactylitis (sausage digit) may be the first manifestation of a spondyloarthropathy in both young children and teenagers. Instead of the joints, the entire finger or toe appears swollen, like a sausage. This is because of swelling around the inflamed tendons as well as the joint. At first, the child is complaining of only a single finger or toe and is initially thought to have injured it. However, on careful examination, periarticular involvement is often evident in multiple joints.

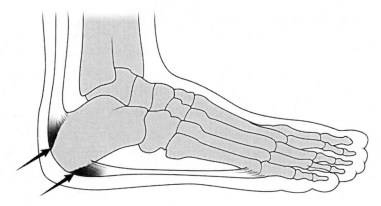

FIG 7-1 *Pain in enthesitis-associated arthritis commonly occurs at the back of the heel (Achilles tendon insertion) or bottom of the heel (plantar fascia insertion).*

Often there is unrecognized inflammation in toes on the same side as the finger that can be found by careful examination. It is also common to find unsuspected wrist involvement on the affected side. These children may be ANA-positive and may have unsuspected eye inflammation. It is important that they be properly screened for eye disease (see Chapter 6).

In teenagers, difficulty bending forward to touch the toes is an additional finding that assists in making this diagnosis. Frequently, physical education instructors have noted that they are not flexible. Sacroiliac joint tenderness is another common finding.

Laboratory findings may not be helpful. Although severe cases may have an elevated sedimentation rate, all tests are often normal in children with mild spondyloarthropathies. HLA B27 is present in about one-half. Rheumatoid factor should never be present. ANA is present in some (see Chapter 22).

Once a child is diagnosed with a spondyloarthropathy, it is important to recognize that this pattern of joint involvement may be associated with a variety of other diseases (discussed later). Many children have a nonspecific spondyloarthropathy, meaning there is no associated condition. However, the associated condition may not become evident until years after the arthritis begins. It's important to be aware of these associations so that the child can be evaluated appropriately. This is particularly true of children who develop recurrent abdominal pain that might be inflammatory bowel disease (IBD); while most children with IBD develop arthritis after their bowel disease is recognized, this is not always the case.

NONSPECIFIC SPONDYLOARTHROPATHIES

Nonspecific spondyloarthropathies, also called enthesitis-associated arthritis or seronegative enthesitis-arthritis syndrome (SEA syndrome), are very common. Children with this diagnosis have the typical findings of a spondyloarthropathy without a recognized associated condition (for example, reactive arthritis). The majority of these children have little if any joint swelling and rarely experience significant problems. But the discomfort and stiffness associated with the enthesitis may result in poor sleep patterns and fatigue. Not uncommonly these children are mislabeled as having fibromyalgia, but it is important to avoid this misdiagnosis, as the proper medications for fibromyalgia are different from those from spondyloarthropathy, as is the prognosis.

Complications of Nonspecific Spondyloarthathies

Complications that do not involve the joints (extra-articular complications) are most common in children who have one of the associated conditions that are discussed below. However, a few specific complications are well recognized to occur in children with nonspecific spondyloarthropathies. Acute anterior uveitis is the most common. This is a painful eye disease involving the front of the eye. Often the eye appears very red, and vision may be affected. This is quite different from the silent eye disease of children with pauciarticular-onset arthritis. Although it may be mistaken for pinkeye (conjunctivitis), it will not respond to antibiotic drops and requires care by an ophthalmologist.

Cardiac involvement in adults with spondyloarthropathies is well recognized. Fortunately, it occurs in only a small number of children. The most common form of cardiac involvement is inflammation of the root of the aorta (the vessel carrying blood out of the heart), which is called aortitis. This inflammation can result in damage to the heart valves and a condition called aortic insufficiency. Children with aortic insufficiency complain of loss of energy and increasing shortness of breath with activity. The condition is easily detected by echocardiography, which is a painless and simple test in which sound waves are bounced off the heart to monitor the motion of the heart valves and muscle. Less frequent complications include involvement of the lungs or kidneys. These cardiac complications have been described in teenagers but are very rare. Most often these complications occur in adults with definite ankylosing spondylitis.

Treatment of Nonspecific Spondyloarthropathies

Treatment for children with spondyloarthropathies must be appropriate to their level of discomfort and their risk of developing severe disease. For example, girls who are at low risk of significant long-term complications infrequently require second-line agents unless they have obvious swollen joints or an elevated erythrocyte sedimentation rate. Of the NSAIDs, diclofenac, nabumetone, piroxicam, etodolac, oxaprozin, and indomethacin are generally more effective for enthesitis than ibuprofen or naproxen. The majority of children can be treated successfully with these NSAIDs. A non-NSAID, sulfasalazine, is often remarkably effective for children with spondyloarthropathies, but it contains sulfur and is associated with an increased frequency of allergic reactions. For children with more severe disease, methotrexate, etanercept, adalimumab, and infliximab all have been used with varying degrees of success (see Chapter 20).

Boys who are HLA B27–positive with a family history of ankylosing spondylitis and/or MRI-documented sacroiliac joint inflammation are at risk of progression to true ankylosing spondylitis as adults. They should be aggressively treated as soon as they are recognized. Early addition of TNF inhibitors and methotrexate is the course most likely to alter their long-term prognosis. It is easier to prevent damage than to repair damage that has occurred.

Physical therapy is important in caring for children who do not fully respond to NSAIDs. The major concern is their progressive loss of flexibility over time. This loss of flexibility can be slowed if not completely prevented by a program of appropriate anti-inflammatory medications, exercises, and strengthening with attention to good posture (see Fig. 7-2). Local inflammatory changes in the wrist may be helped by the use of wrist splints to protect against subluxation and to reduce discomfort. For children with plantar fascia insertion pain or heel spurs, the use of gel-filled heel cups in the shoe may provide substantial relief.

Surgery is rarely necessary for children with spondyloarthropathy. In the small subgroup of children with severe disease, it may become necessary to replace a damaged hip. Occasionally, children develop severe wrist arthritis and may require surgical fusion. Chronic active arthritis may require a synovectomy. With proper physical therapy, it is uncommon for children to need tendon releases.

Prognosis for Children with Nonspecific Spondyloarthropathy

The majority of children with spondyloarthropathies do well. When considering prognosis, it is important to consider gender, whether the child is positive or

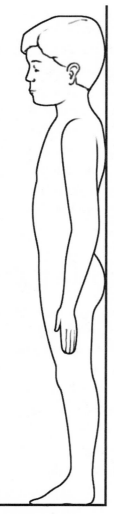

FIG 7-2 *Children should practice good posture by standing with their heels, buttocks, shoulders, and back of the head flat against the wall.*

negative for HLA B27, and whether the sedimentation rate is elevated or normal. Girls who are HLA B27–negative with a normal sedimentation rate do well in the long run but may have recurrent complaints. Many require NSAIDs on a consistent basis, especially in the wintertime, but it is rare for this illness to have a major negative impact on their lives. Most of these children have recurrent enthesitis, but swollen joints are rare. HLA B27–positive girls with a normal sedimentation rate tend to have a higher frequency of complaints and more frequently recurring disease than girls who are HLA B27–negative, but again have a good long-term prognosis.

Girls who have an elevated sedimentation rate or recurrent joint swelling are more worrisome. Some of these girls have significant arthritis that will require continuing care and may necessitate the use of sulfasalazine, TNF inhibitors, or other second-line drugs. Nonetheless, they should be able to manage all everyday activities without problem. The prognosis is a little more guarded for the girls who have elevated sedimentation rates and swollen joints and are HLA B27–positive. This group is more likely to require TNF inhibitors and to have problems that persist into adulthood. However, with proper care they should still have a very acceptable outcome and enjoy a full life.

Most HLA B27–negative boys with a nonspecific spondyloarthropathy also do well. However, their complaints tend to be more frequent and more severe than the complaints of HLA B27–negative girls. They also tend to have more persistent problems with heel pain and back pain. This group may require long-term medication and often TNF inhibitors. They generally function well as adults but are typically excluded from the armed forces and emergency services because of their lack of flexibility.

Boys with an elevated sedimentation rate and swollen joints are at greater risk of an unsatisfactory outcome. They may have more difficulty over the long term and often require TNF inhibitors. Although their outcome is usually quite acceptable, there are HLA B27–negative boys whose arthritis persists into adulthood. Nonetheless, most have jobs and families and are not limited by their arthritis, with the exception of athletic activities and occupational limitations as above.

There are two distinct groups of HLA B27–positive boys. Some have normal sedimentation rates, no swollen joints, and only mild complaints. It appears that they have only minimal genetic predisposition toward arthritis (see Chapter 22). Like the others in this group, these children do well. Boys who are HLA B27–positive and have swollen joints with an elevated ESR are at greater risk. Some will go on to develop definite ankylosing spondylitis or another associated condition (see the next sections).

JUVENILE ANKYLOSING SPONDYLITIS AND ANKYLOSING SPONDYLITIS

Virtually all adult men with ankylosing spondylitis (AS), which is chronic inflammation of the spine and sacroiliac joints, are positive for the genetic marker HLA B27–positive, but we do not know how many boys who are positive for HLA B27 will never develop AS. Most individuals with AS do not fulfill criteria for the diagnosis until after they reach thirty years of age, and it is difficult to keep track of HLA B27–positive teenagers for the fifteen years or more of follow-up needed to answer that question. Therefore, I do not recommend diagnosing every boy who is positive for HLA B27 and has a spondyloarthropathy as having juvenile ankylosing spondylitis (JAS). Not only does it cause undue worry for many parents, but it may also make life and health insurance difficult to obtain. Although some will develop AS, not all will, and labeling them is unnecessary. However, an HLA B27–positive boy who has swollen joints and an elevated sedimentation rate is at risk of progressing to definite AS and certainly should be treated aggressively.

Occasionally, I see HLA B27–positive teenage boys who have obvious sacroiliac joint involvement on their X-rays and can be labeled definitively as having AS (a certain amount of sacroiliac involvement is the diagnostic criterion for AS). However, this is uncommon. I am concerned if there is evidence of sacroiliitis on MRI; these children should be treated more aggressively even though we aren't sure they will ultimately be diagnosed with AS.

REACTIVE ARTHRITIS: INFECTION-ASSOCIATED ARTHRITIS AND REITER'S SYNDROME

Reactive or infection-associated arthritis is a type of spondyloarthropathy brought on by infection. Reiter's syndrome is a special case of infection-associated arthritis with a particular set of systems (discussed later). Affected children are often very ill, with fever, rash, and arthritis. Sometimes the arthritis is in only one large joint, but at other times it may be widespread, affecting many joints both large and small. It was originally termed "reactive arthritis" because the arthritis frequently begins shortly after a significant viral or bacterial infection. The name was changed to infection-associated arthritis to remind physicians that in some cases the infection is still present and may require treatment.

The most common infectious agents that cause these forms of arthritis are bacteria (shigella, salmonella, neisseria, and chlamydia) and viruses (especially parvovirus B19). The arthritis associated with Lyme disease is also a form of infection-associated arthritis. Mild and brief arthritis following a variety of infections is very common. Once the episode has passed, most children recover completely. A typical episode of infection-associated arthritis resolves in three to six weeks. However, some children develop arthritis that lasts for a longer period. If the arthritis persists for a year or more, then it is considered arthritis that was initiated by an infection, but it is no longer considered reactive or infection-associated arthritis.

Although many children with infection-associated arthritis look very ill at the beginning, the majority of children recover completely. Some are initially misdiagnosed as having systemic-onset arthritis, but the fever pattern and rash of reactive arthritis and systemic-onset arthritis are different. Recurrences of reactive arthritis are rare (if the underlying infection has resolved), but there are children with a substantial genetic predisposition to arthritis who develop repeated episodes of arthritis following exposure to different infectious agents.

Complications of Reactive Arthritis

Since, by definition, infection-associated arthritis resolves within a year of onset, long-term complications are infrequent. There may be complications related to the initial infection, but most children recover fully and do well.

Reiter's syndrome, as noted previously, is a special case of reactive arthritis. It is distinguished from other cases of reactive arthritis by the occurrence of arthritis, urethritis (irritation of the urinary tract), and conjunctivitis. Children with Reiter's syndrome sometimes have rashes, particularly on their hands and feet. They may also have severe, painful acute anterior uveitis. When evaluating a child for the diagnosis of Reiter's syndrome, it is important to remember that the arthritis, urethritis, and conjunctivitis do not all have to be present on the same day. They may occur one after the other without ever overlapping in time. Although Reiter's syndrome with all of the findings is common in adults, it is rare in childhood.

Treatment of Reactive Arthritis

The most important step in the treatment for children with any kind of infection-associated arthritis involves making sure the infection is properly treated. Once it is clear that the infection associated with the arthritis is no longer active, these children should be treated just like other children with spondyloarthropathies. Most respond well to NSAIDs. In most cases, the arthritis resolves completely over a period of a few months. TNF inhibitors are sometimes required, while other children benefit from the addition of sulfasalazine. Intra-articular injection of corticosteroids may be useful if only one joint remains troublesome after the infection has been fully treated, but oral corticosteroids are rarely necessary.

Physical therapy to maintain strength and range of motion is often necessary during the acute phase of the disease. Surgery should not be necessary for a child with infection-associated arthritis unless it is required to treat the infection.

Prognosis for Children with Reactive Arthritis

Once the infection is properly treated and has resolved, the long-term prognosis for children with infection-associated arthritis is very good. Occasionally, children have recurrent episodes of arthritis with subsequent infections. Rarely children may have an episode of infection-associated arthritis, recover, and then develop persistent spondyloarthropathy years later.

PSORIATIC ARTHRITIS

Psoriatic arthritis is another spondyloarthropathy that requires special attention. Pediatric rheumatologists continue to debate exactly who belongs in this group, since a child does not have to have psoriasis to have psoriatic arthritis, and children might have another form of arthritis and coincidentally have psoriasis. It is called psoriatic arthritis because over the course of as much as ten to fifteen years, many children who have this type of arthritis will develop psoriasis. Whether they eventually develop psoriasis or not, what's most important is that in children diagnosed with this condition, their disease behaves like the arthritis associated with psoriasis and responds to the same medications.

There are varied criteria for the diagnosis of psoriatic arthritis. They require that the child have arthritis plus dactylitis or changes in the fingernails of a type often seen in children with psoriasis (onycholysis), as well as a close relative with psoriasis. Some physicians argue over how close the relative must be and how sure you need be that the relative has psoriasis. What is most important is that this arthritis has a characteristic appearance and behavior. If a child presents with dactylitis or obvious swollen tendons, it is most likely psoriatic arthritis.

The group of children with psoriatic arthritis is divided into two main subgroups. One group is made up of young children, mostly girls, who are often ANA-positive and may have pauciarticular-onset disease. These children often have an elevated sedimentation rates or low hemoglobin. Many of these children start with a swollen finger or toe (dactylitis). The other group consists of older children with more typical polyarticular-onset disease.

Though young children with this form of arthritis, those in the first subgroup, may look just like children with pauciarticular-onset arthritis, they need to be treated more aggressively. Most often they are girls, but there are some boys in this group. Frequently they will have an elevated sedimentation rate or low hemoglobin. Interestingly, they are often ANA-positive and as much at risk of eye disease as the true pauciarticular-onset children. Some will have a family history of psoriasis. The dactylitis may occur at the same time as the arthritis appears, or it may have appeared months before and have already cleared up by the time a knee is affected.

Despite the fact that only a few joints are affected at the beginning, over time the children in this first group often develop polyarticular disease. A typical child might have had a swollen toe at eighteen months that rapidly improved, then a swollen knee at thirty-six months that improved over six months, then swollen wrists at age six that are still causing trouble at age twelve. The key to obtaining a good outcome for these children is aggressive therapy to bring their disease under control. They are often more difficult to bring under control with NSAIDs, and their disease recurs much more frequently. The TNF inhibitors, such as etanercept and adalimumab, are very effective in this group and should be considered early in the therapy of children who are not responding adequately to NSAIDs. Once the disease is under control, the children typically need prolonged therapy with a medication such as sulfasalazine.

In the second subgroup of children with psoriatic arthritis, children who are older (often between twelve and sixteen years) at disease onset, again girls are more common than boys. Often they give no history of earlier problems. Their problems may begin with a swollen finger or toe, and they are almost invariably thought to have suffered recurrent athletic injuries. Some present with a swollen wrist without evidence of any other joint involvement. They often have an elevated sedimentation rate, and about half have a family history of psoriasis. Sometimes the arthritis is difficult to control. In other children it seems to come under control easily, but it keeps coming back. It is unlikely that this form of arthritis is ever truly gone. A significant number of these children develop widespread arthritis over time. However, most respond well to aggressive therapy. As with all forms of arthritis in childhood, early intervention is essential to prevent the accumulation of significant long-term joint damage. Since it frequently recurs, continued follow-up even when the child seems well is also important so that subtle signs of disease progression can be detected before permanent damage occurs.

Complications of Psoriatic Arthritis

The primary complications of psoriatic arthritis are related to recurrent arthritis. Some children develop significant joint damage over the course of their disease. Serious eye involvement can occur in young children, and children with ANA-positive psoriatic arthritis must be monitored just as carefully as children with ANA-positive pauciarticular-onset JA. Fortunately, eye involvement is less common in teenagers but still possible. Persistent wrist and finger involvement is often prominent. In some children this seems to be the only evidence of disease. However, children may begin with only wrist involvement but years later develop problems in other joints. Elbow, neck, and jaw involvement is more common in children with this form of arthritis and must be looked for. However, hips, knees, ankles, and toes may also be involved. Because the arthritis can become widespread, it is important to do everything possible to bring it under control quickly and, if possible, to prevent it from returning.

Treatment of Psoriatic Arthritis

Initial treatment for this group is the same as the treatment for other children with spondyloarthropathies. Diclofenac, nabumetone, piroxicam, etodolac, oxaprozin, and indomethacin are generally more effective for enthesitis than ibuprofen or naproxen. I am much quicker to use sulfasalazine and TNF inhibitors such as etanercept and adalimumab for children in this group, as the TNF inhibitors act fast and provide superior relief, and studies have suggested that children who are taking sulfasalazine as well are likely to have a better long-term outcome than children taking TNF inhibitors alone. I have cared for a number of children who did very well for several years on sulfasalazine, but then had recurrent disease within a few months of stopping the drug. As a result, in the absence of side effects, I continue sulfasalazine as long as possible. While problems with sulfasalazine most often occur at the beginning of treatment, children on long-term therapy with sulfasalazine or TNF inhibitors (or any other medication) require routine monitoring of their laboratory tests (see Chapter 20).

Methotrexate is often used in the treatment of children with psoriatic arthritis. It is effective, both alone and in combination with TNF inhibitors. However, its onset of action is slower than the TNF inhibitors and it has additional side effects. I tend to reserve methotrexate for children with severe disease who are not responding adequately to TNF inhibitors alone. Thalidomide has been effective in children who have failed all other therapies, but its use requires particular precautions (see Chapter 20 for more details). Except for occasional intra-articular injections, corticosteroids are rarely necessary and should be avoided if at all possible.

Physical therapy plays an important role in maintaining strength and range of motion for these children. Since this form of arthritis has a propensity to involve the wrists and fingers, occupational therapy is often an important part of their care as well.

Surgery is rarely necessary for children with psoriatic arthritis. For children with severe disease it may be necessary to replace a damaged hip. Occasionally, children develop severe, painful wrist arthritis that may require surgical fusion. With proper physical therapy it is uncommon for children to need tendon releases or any other surgical procedures.

Prognosis for Children with Psoriatic Arthritis

The long-term prognosis for children with psoriatic arthritis is more guarded than for children with a nonspecific spondyloarthropathy or typical pauciarticular-onset JA. Young children who have only dactylitis that resolves quickly may develop arthritis in other joints years later. Now that use of TNF inhibitors is routine, however, with aggressive therapy and careful monitoring most children with psoriatic arthritis will have a very acceptable, if not perfect, outcome.

ARTHRITIS ASSOCIATED WITH GASTROINTESTINAL COMPLAINTS

Ulcerative colitis and regional enteritis are collectively referred to as inflammatory bowel disease (IBD). It is well known that some children with these diseases have arthritis that typically takes the form of a spondyloarthropathy and which may become evident before the IBD. Studies have demonstrated that many individuals with spondyloarthropathy have an unusual appearance to their gastrointestinal mucosa (lining). Exactly how this relates to developing arthritis is uncertain.

Children with IBD are often on strong immunosuppressive medications for the IBD. They also may be receiving corticosteroids. In most cases the therapy for their IBD is sufficient to control their arthritis. However, occasionally, children require NSAIDs in addition to the therapy for their IBD. Infliximab and adalimumab are beneficial for children who don't respond to NSAIDs.

In evaluating a child with a spondyloarthropathy who has gastrointestinal complaints, testing for the antibody pANCA may speed recognition of the child with IBD. Either of two skin findings, erythema nodosum (large, tender, painful, red or purplish bumps over the shins) or pyoderma gangrenosum (large areas of skin breakdown with weeping sores), in a child with a spondyloarthropathy should spark careful consideration for possible IBD. Many of the children with arthritis and IBD are HLA B27–positive. Children with IBD who are HLA B27–positive are more likely to have significant and persistent arthritis than those who are HLA B27–negative.

In addition to IBD, children who have abdominal pain, rash, and arthritis might have reactive arthritis, Henoch-Schoenlein purpura, Kawasaki disease, polyarteritis nodosa, dermatomyositis, systemic lupus erythematosus, or other vasculitic diseases, among other possible conditions. Most often the correct diagnosis is evident, but I have seen children with IBD initially misdiagnosed with these illnesses, and vice versa.

Celiac disease (gluten-sensitive enteropathy) is another gastrointestinal disease associated with arthritic complaints that typically takes the form of a spondyloarthropathy. Celiac disease most often begins with poor growth during the first years of life. However, celiac disease is being increasingly recognized in teenagers with nonspecific joint complaints or spondyloarthropathies and chronic upset stomachs. When questioned, many of these children complain of disliking pasta, pizza, and other high-gluten foods. A definite diagnosis of celiac disease requires characteristic findings on a biopsy of the small intestine, but the diagnosis is strongly suggested by the presence of antiendomysial antibodies (IgA antitissue transglutaminase) in the blood. Treatment for celiac disease is a gluten-free diet. With this the arthritic complaints will normally subside. Untreated celiac disease is associated with a number of autoimmune conditions, including thyroiditis (inflammation of the thyroid gland), and may be associated with a positive ANA.

Nonspecific arthritic complaints may also be seen in children who have recovered from a severe insult to the gastrointestinal tract. The most common example is children who suffered necrotizing enterocolitis (severe inflammation of the lining of the intestines) during the neonatal period.

Since there are a variety of conditions that both affect the gastrointestinal tract and cause arthritis, it is natural to wonder how the two problems are associated. There are no studies that answer this question to everyone's satisfaction. It appears that an intestinal tract that is damaged or otherwise "different" may allow elements from the diet to get into the bloodstream. In some people (perhaps because of genetic predisposition), these elements may reach the joints and initiate arthritis. If the damage to the intestinal tract can be corrected, the arthritis may go away. This association has led to the hope that dietary changes may relieve the arthritis. This is true for children with celiac disease who improve if they avoid foods containing gluten. However, it does not appear to be true for other conditions (see Chapter 21).

One special situation that deserves attention is the child with a complaint of severe abdominal pain, fever, arthritis, and limp. Though most children with appendicitis develop fever and severe abdominal pain and are promptly diagnosed, if a child has been ill with severe abdominal pain and develops a limp on the right side, the physician should remember to consider the possibility of undiagnosed appendicitis.

Complications of Arthritis Associated with Gastrointestinal Complaints

The long-term complications of children with IBD are primarily related to their gastrointestinal disease and its treatment and are not discussed here.

Complications of the arthritis of IBD are similar to those of children with spondyloarthropathy. With the exception of hip and sacroiliac joint involvement, the arthritis rarely is of long-term significance.

Treatment of Arthritis Associated with Gastrointestinal Complaints

Adalimumab has recently been approved as therapy for inflammatory bowel disease. This agent is extremely effective for the arthritis of IBD as well as for the disease itself. Use of adalimumab is increasing, as there is growing hesitation on the part of gastroenterologists to use NSAIDs in children with inflammatory bowel disease because of the medications' propensity to cause gastrointestinal side effects.

Physical and occupational therapy for these children is the same as for other children with other spondyloarthropathies.

MISCELLANEOUS CONDITIONS RELATED TO SPONDYLOARTHROPATHIES

Hypogammaglobulinemia-Associated Problems

IgA deficiency. IgA deficiency is a low level of immunoglobulin A (see Chapter 22). Children with IgA deficiency develop rheumatic diseases much more frequently than the normal population. While this often takes the form of a spondyloarthropathy, studies have shown an increased frequency of children with IgA deficiency in virtually every rheumatic disease.

There are two important problems to be aware of regarding a child who is recognized to have IgA deficiency. The first is to recognize that this is a permanent condition that makes recurrent arthritis more likely, even in a child who otherwise appears to have pauciarticular-onset disease. The second problem is that individuals who are IgA-deficient are vulnerable to transfusion reactions. These are not due to incompatibility with the transfused red blood cells but are the result of a reaction to the IgA in the serum transfused with the red blood cells. Routine laboratory cross-typing will not detect this. Parents of children who are IgA-deficient should be sure that they inform any treating physician of this condition. A clue to the presence of IgA deficiency is a strong history of recurrent ear infections or similar problems. However, many children who have had lots of ear infections do not have any identified abnormality.

Common variable hypogammaglobulinemia. This is a condition in which children with immature immune systems do not have fully normal levels of immunoglobulin. Children from three to seven years of age who limp whenever they have a viral infection often have low immunoglobulin levels. On evaluation they often have a very mild degree of periarticular pain and no other obvious findings. The complaints typically disappear in a day or a few days, when the infection has resolved. However, the limp or other joint pains may recur with subsequent infections. I have seen a number of children with six, seven, or even eight such episodes.

Routine laboratory evaluation of these children is usually completely normal. When serum immunoglobulin levels are measured, the children have values that would clearly be abnormal for an adult but are considered at the low end of normal for their age, so they are not officially immunodeficient. As these children's immune system matures, the immunoglobulin levels rise and the problem ceases. No detailed reports of the long-term outcome for these children are available. None that I have cared for has developed significant rheumatic disease, though many have been misdiagnosed as having JA.

Children with definite common variable hypogammaglobulinemia and IgG subclass deficiencies (low immunoglobulin levels of varying specific types) may also have an increased incidence of arthritis. The arthritis these children get also generally follows the pattern of a spondyloarthropathy. Many investigators feel that this situation is similar to the situation for children with abnormal gastrointestinal tracts. In children with mild immune deficiencies, proteins or other molecules that are normally kept out of the body by the immune system are able to get in and cause mild arthritis. In most children these episodes are short-lived and without serious complications, but there are exceptions. In addition, it is important to recognize that the defect in their immune systems leaves them vulnerable to bone or joint infections.

Children with more severe forms of immunodeficiency are occasionally found to have arthritis. For these children, the immune deficiency and the resulting infections are usually a more significant problem than the arthritis. However, these children may benefit from treatment with NSAIDs. Often the underlying immunodeficiency is treated with intravenous immunoglobulin (IV IgG), and this leads to resolution of the arthritis as well.

Post-Streptococcal Reactive Arthritis and Rheumatic Fever

Post-streptococcal reactive arthritis is another form of infection-associated arthritis. It differs in that we know this form of infection-associated arthritis is initiated by a group A streptococcal infection. Post-streptococcal reactive arthritis behaves just like the other forms of infection-associated arthritis. Sometimes the arthritis is in a single large joint such as the hip, and at other times it can affect multiple joints.

There is a lot of confusion regarding the relationship of post-streptococcal reactive arthritis to acute rheumatic fever. Since acute rheumatic fever is associated with possible damage to the heart and requires penicillin prophylaxis, this is an area of great concern. Acute rheumatic fever is defined according to the Jones criteria (see box). Children who develop a nonmigratory (not moving from joint to joint) arthritis after a streptococcal infection do not fulfill these criteria. As a result, many physicians do not treat these children with penicillin prophylaxis. However, some of these children have gone on to develop heart damage of rheumatic fever following a later streptococcal infection.

Jones Criteria for the Diagnosis of Acute Rheumatic Fever

Major criteria

- Carditis (inflammation of the heart valves or muscle)
- Migratory polyarticular arthritis (swollen and tender joints with involvement shifting from one joint to another)
- Sydenham's chorea (a type of uncontrollable movements)
- Subcutaneous nodules (bumps under the skin)
- Erythema marginatum (a red rash with dramatic red outlines)

Minor criteria

- Raised CRP, ESR, or leukocytes (laboratory results)
- Arthralgia (joint pain without swelling or limitation)
- Fever

The diagnosis of acute rheumatic fever requires two major criteria, or one major and two minor criteria, and evidence of a recent streptococcal infection.

Since no large-scale studies have been carried out to determine how much risk there is for children with post-streptococcal reactive arthritis who do not fulfill the Jones criteria, there is no definite answer regarding penicillin prophylaxis for these children. In families where there is a history of acute rheumatic fever or in children where the arthritis associated with the streptococcal infection was severe, I prefer to treat with penicillin prophylaxis to prevent recurrences and reduce the risk of future rheumatic fever-related heart damage. However, this must be balanced against the risks of penicillin allergy and the appearance of bacteria that are resistant to penicillin.

The arthritis in children with post-streptococcal reactive arthritis is usually short-lived and treated with NSAIDs, just like other forms of spondyloarthropathy. The prognosis is primarily related to heart involvement. Children with the severe inflammation of the heart seen in acute rheumatic fever are at risk of permanent heart damage or even death and should be under the care of a cardiologist.

8

Lyme Disease

Lyme disease is a chronic infection by the bacterium *Borrelia burgdorferi*, which is carried by mammals such as deer and deer mice and spread by very small deer ticks (*Ixodes scapularis*). The ticks bite an infected animal and pick up the spirochete with their blood meal. They then transfer the spirochete to people or animals they feed on, infecting them with Lyme disease.

Lyme disease in humans is often only an acute flu-like illness. However, some adults and children develop rash and arthritis. The key to understanding Lyme arthritis in children is to recognize that it is in many ways a typical infection-associated arthritis. The major difference is that Lyme disease follows a much more protracted course. Typical infection-associated arthritis develops within a few weeks of the original illness. The fever and rash of Lyme disease also occur early. However, the arthritis of Lyme disease usually does not appear until two to four months or more after the initial infection, and if it is no longer tick season, parents and physicians may not be thinking of Lyme as a potential cause of arthritis.

In children the flu-like symptoms of early Lyme disease are often dismissed as a virus. The child may develop the characteristic rash a few weeks after the original illness. This is most often a circle the size of a quarter, sometimes much bigger. The outer edge of the circle is red and inflamed-looking, while the center of the circle is usually pale. Anyone with such a rash should be tested and treated for Lyme disease (though there are other illnesses that may produce a similar rash). Children do not usually have arthritis when the rash first appears. However, the rash can recur later in the illness when the child does have arthritis.

A number of nonspecific symptoms, such as headaches, are often seen at the beginning of Lyme disease. Their significance is uncertain. While the disease can involve the nervous system in some children, most children with headaches do not have Lyme. Bell's palsy, one symptom of Lyme disease (though there are many other possible causes), is an irritation of the facial nerve that is responsible for moving one side of the face. If this nerve is not functioning properly, the child may have difficulty or be unable to open the mouth, smile, or close the eye tightly on the involved side.

Lyme arthritis usually begins dramatically. It can affect any large or small joint and often suddenly affects many joints, though some children with Lyme present with only a single swollen joint. Lyme-infected children are often in significant pain. This is very different from typical childhood arthritis, which comes on gradually. In addition, like other forms of infection-associated arthritis, Lyme arthritis can begin in the hip (though it does not cause dactylitis). Children with Lyme disease who have gone untreated for a long period of time may have recurrent episodes of joint swelling. This most often takes the form of recurrent knee swelling, which may have been dismissed as an athletic injury or sprain.

Since the arthritic symptoms develop months after the initial tick bite, children with the arthritis of Lyme disease are easily diagnosed only if the physician remembers to check a Lyme titer. However, it is important to remember that children with other serious illness that can cause arthritis may also have been exposed to Lyme in the past and have a positive titer even though Lyme is not the explanation for their symptoms. At the same time, children who already have juvenile arthritis, live in or have visited an area where Lyme disease is endemic, and have unexpectedly developed a dramatic worsening of their symptoms may have acquired a Lyme infection and should be tested. Because the children I follow have chronic arthritis, I systematically check Lyme titers in the fall each year.

DIFFERENTIAL DIAGNOSIS OF LYME DISEASE

Lyme disease is a typical infection-associated or reactive arthritis. As a result, it can be confused with other infection-associated types of arthritis. The key differences in children with arthritis due to Lyme disease are the absence of a recent infection (most children develop infection-associated arthritis ten to fourteen days following a recognized illness) and the presence of a positive Lyme titer.

Systemic lupus erythematosus and other forms of collagen vascular disease may also begin with the rapid onset of arthritis involving the large and small joints. The key to distinguishing these diseases is their different clinical appearance and use of appropriate laboratory testing. In areas where there is a high frequency of exposure to Lyme disease, the situation may be complicated by a positive Lyme test in a child who is suffering from another illness. All children with positive Lyme tests should be treated for Lyme disease, but if there is not a quick and dramatic response, the physician should investigate other possible causes of the child's symptoms.

There is much debate about the occurrence of Lyme disease in children who do not have positive titers (see Chapter 22). Most of this debate stems from the period when Lyme testing was not well standardized. At present, it is extremely unlikely that a child with a negative Lyme titer has the disease. While it is always possible for the laboratory to make a mistake in reporting a result, this can be easily resolved in a suspicious situation by simply repeating the test, perhaps using a different laboratory.

LABORATORY FINDINGS IN LYME DISEASE

Children with Lyme disease almost invariably have a positive Lyme titer and a positive Western blot (see Chapter 22). In addition, they have elevated ESRs and white blood cell counts. While the elevated white blood cell count and ESR are commonly present in children with polyarticular-onset arthritis, they are infrequent in children with pauciarticular-onset disease. Some children with Lyme disease have positive tests for antinuclear antibody (ANA). They should not have rheumatoid factor (RF), antibodies to double-stranded DNA, or complement abnormalities.

The Lyme titer and Western blot are the standard tests; other tests exist but are not as reliable. While a child with a high suspicion for Lyme disease and a positive ELISA but negative Western blot may deserve two weeks of antibiotics, if symptoms persist it is unwise to continue treatment. Such children need a complete and thorough evaluation for other possible causes of their symptoms.

COMPLICATIONS OF LYME DISEASE

Fortunately, serious complications of Lyme disease are rare. The vast majority of children with Lyme-related arthritis recover promptly (within a few weeks) and completely with treatment. In children with Lyme who have large numbers of bands on their Western blot (e.g., nine or more), it is likely the infection has been present for a prolonged period. Some of these children will have continuing arthritis after the first thirty days of antibiotics. It is important to recognize that, like other causes of infection-associated arthritis, Lyme tends to provoke symptoms in those who have an underlying predisposition to arthritis. If the arthritis persists after appropriate treatment for Lyme disease, the emphasis must be on treatment of the arthritis, not continued antibiotics. For any child whose arthritis persists after a year we must assume that Lyme provoked an underlying arthritic disease; it is that underlying disease that must be treated.

Some argue that Lyme produces many chronic symptoms in children, including attention deficit disorder and other unexplained conditions. It is important to recognize that Lyme disease is common. Therefore it will be found in a significant number of children with a wide variety of coincidental problems that are unrelated to Lyme disease. The issue seems clear-cut: if the child's problems resolve with treatment, they were due to the Lyme disease, but if the problems are not related to Lyme, months or even years of antibiotics are unlikely to provide real relief.

Another possible complication of Lyme disease is the Jarisch-Herxheimer reaction, which occurs when a dose of antibiotic is given to a patient with a large number of bacteria in his or her system and the bacteria release their contents into the bloodstream, causing an acute toxic reaction with fever, rash, and severe malaise. However, I have never seen this reaction in a child under my care.

TREATMENT OF LYME DISEASE

Optimal treatment for Lyme disease is dependent on the age of the child, the manifestations of the disease, and whether the child has any allergies to drugs. Young children are typically treated with amoxicillin, while children over the age of ten are typically treated with doxycycline. Doxycycline is not used in younger children because it will become incorporated in the enamel of developing teeth and may cause a permanent grayish stain. Some physicians feel it is acceptable to use doxycycline in children as young as eight years of age if the adult teeth appear to be fully formed in the gums. In children who are allergic to these drugs, consideration may be given to cephalosporins or erythromycin derivatives. This should be discussed carefully with your physician because these drugs differ in how well they reach the central nervous system.

The duration of therapy for Lyme disease also depends on the manifestations of disease. The majority of the medical community is in agreement with the recommendations shown in the box.

One of the least settled questions in the treatment of Lyme disease is the response to children found with an embedded deer tick. The correct answer is to obtain a Lyme titer. It will not reflect infection from the tick just found, but may indicate that there is a preexisting infection that requires treatment. If this titer is negative, it needs to be repeated in six weeks to determine whether it has turned positive. If it has, the child should be treated appropriately.

Some physicians recommend an alternative approach. If a child is found with an embedded tick, a Lyme titer is performed, but two weeks of oral antibiotic therapy are begun immediately. If the titer is negative, treatment is stopped at two weeks. If the titer is positive, then treatment is continued for an additional week. It has been shown that this may prevent Lyme infections and is more cost-effective than repeated testing. One new study suggests one day of treatment may work as well as two weeks. However, if a child lives in an area where Lyme is common, how often are we going to treat him or her? There is no answer to this question that everyone agrees with. Often parents will bring a tick to the physician to have the tick tested for Lyme disease. This is useless because of the small size of the deer tick. If the child had one tick that the parents found, there is a significant chance the child had other ticks that the parents didn't find. The child must be tested, not the tick.

Unfortunately, it is difficult to tell if a child who has had Lyme disease in the past has a new infection. The child's titer will be positive from the previous infection, and it is virtually impossible to culture the spirochete from tissues to prove an infection is present. Currently there is no vaccine against Lyme; an earlier vaccine was withdrawn from the market because it had side effects and did not guarantee protection from future infection.

Duration of Antibiotic Therapy for Lyme Disease

- Children with a positive test for Lyme disease in the absence of arthritis or neurologic symptoms should be treated with 21 days of an appropriate antibiotic.
- If a child has arthritis, 30 days of antibiotic therapy are recommended. For a possible bacterial infection of the joint, the antibiotic may be started intravenously and switched to oral only after bacterial infection has been excluded. To control the inflammatory response in the joint, the child should also be treated with NSAIDs for as long as the arthritis continues.
- Children with neurologic manifestations of Lyme disease also require 30 days of antibiotic therapy; many physicians prefer to begin with intravenous therapy. Further treatment of children with neurologic manifestations that have not completely resolved after 30 days of intravenous therapy will depend on the nature of the symptoms and the degree of improvement that has occurred.
- Children who have arthritis that has not fully resolved with 30 days of oral therapy represent a challenge. For children who have only a moderate number of bands on the Western blot, I recommend a month of continued NSAID therapy. Children with

a large number of bands on the Western blot may have had Lyme-associated arthritis for a long time before it was recognized; for them I recommend an additional 30 days (no more) of intravenous antibiotic therapy to ensure that the Lyme has been adequately treated, followed by NSAIDs.

In my patients, I periodically monitor the Lyme titer and Western blot. During the first few months after diagnosis and treatment, both the Lyme titer and the number of Western blot positive bands may increase. This represents "immunologic recruitment" (the immune response is gathering strength over time), not continued infection. After six or more months, the Lyme titer should begin to decrease. The number of positive bands on the Western blot may not. If a child develops signs of possible repeat infection a year or more after initial treatment, I will compare the results with those found six months after the initial treatment (to account for the immunologic recruitment). If the response is stronger, I will re-treat with oral antibiotics.

There are some physicians who believe that Lyme is a more chronic infection and may require years of therapy. There is no convincing evidence that they are correct, and prolonged antibiotic therapy has been associated with serious side effects.

9

Systemic Lupus Erythematosus

Systemic lupus erythematosus (SLE) is a complex autoimmune disease that most often affects teenage girls and young adult women. Less frequently, SLE occurs in both older and younger individuals and in boys. SLE often begins with fevers, rash, joint pains, and fatigue. Although these symptoms are worrisome, it is the ability of SLE to affect many different internal organs (brain, heart, lungs, muscles, kidneys, skin, joints, liver, or intestine) that makes this a serious illness. It is important that children who have SLE be promptly recognized so that they can be treated and internal organ damage prevented whenever possible.

The key to understanding SLE is to recognize that the disease begins with a breakdown in regulation of the immune system. In a normal immune response, the immune system identifies an invader and mounts a response against it using many different systems. Once the invader has been controlled, the system turns off and everything goes back to normal. In children with SLE, however, the immune system is constantly activated. Whenever the areas damaged by SLE are examined, doctors find the type of damage they would expect if there had been a serious infection.

We are beginning to understand more about why the immune system fails to turn off in children with SLE, but we do not understand why certain children with the disease develop one set of problems and other children develop completely different problems. In animal models, genetics seem to be an important factor that determines which problems develop.

DIAGNOSIS: WHEN TO SUSPECT SLE

SLE most often affects girls in the teenage years, but it may affect boys and girls at any age. Although a butterfly-shaped rash on the face is considered a characteristic feature of the disease, it is found in only one-third of children when they first come to the doctor's office. Since many doctors do not think of SLE unless they see the butterfly rash, many children have symptoms of SLE for months before the proper diagnosis is made. The key to a prompt diagnosis of SLE is for primary-care physicians to consider this diagnosis whenever they are evaluating children who appear chronically ill or have unexplained damage in organs that are frequently affected by SLE, such as the kidneys.

Many physicians are confused by the American College of Rheumatology criteria for a definite diagnosis of SLE (see box). The criteria were written to help distinguish SLE from other diseases; they are not the most frequent symptoms. The three most common symptoms of SLE are fever, a chronic complaint of not feeling well (malaise), and arthritis of the small joints of the hands and feet.

Parents and physicians must consider SLE whenever a child is not doing well. For very young children who are failing to thrive, there is a standard evaluation to look for problems such as cystic fibrosis and hypothyroidism. Physicians also need a standard workup for older children who are failing to thrive. Although SLE is only one of many possible causes, it is important to include ANA testing in this evaluation. Many diseases may be associated with a positive ANA test in children and teenagers (see Chapter 22). However, SLE should be excluded when evaluating any child with a positive test. A negative test for ANA makes SLE very unlikely.

American College of Rheumatology Criteria for a Diagnosis of Definite SLE

1. Malar rash: a red rash over the cheeks (often crossing over the nose)
2. Discoid rash: a scaly red rash (uncommon in children)
3. Photosensitivity: burns easily in sun, rashes and sensitivity to light
4. Mucosal ulcers: sores in the mouth or nose
5. Serositis: inflammation of the lining of the chest or abdomen, producing pain
6. Arthritis: pain swelling or limitation of motion of a joint
7. Renal involvement: abnormalities on the urine tests or blood tests
8. Neurologic involvement: problems with seizures or difficulty thinking normally
9. Hematologic involvement: abnormalities of the red cells, white cells, or platelets
10. Immunologic disorder: abnormal blood tests characteristic of SLE
11. Antinuclear antibodies

A child is considered to have definite SLE if he or she has any four of the eleven criteria.

Although the onset of SLE typically occurs between the ages of twelve and twenty-five years in most patients, it can occur in children as young as three. The incidence of SLE varies by sex and race, but from my experience I find that among girls between nine and nineteen it occurs most frequently in Asians and next most frequently in African Americans, followed by Hispanics and whites. The number of affected boys is much, much smaller. Relatives of someone with SLE are at greater risk of developing SLE than the rest of the population.

Although chronic failure to thrive is the most common presentation in children, SLE can also begin in many other ways. Chronic swelling of the hands and feet, easy bruising, joint pains, abnormal urine tests, photosensitivity, seizures, altered personality and depression, and even altered school performance all may be initial findings. However, it is important to remember that these are nonspecific symptoms that may occur in many different illnesses.

Some children with SLE reach my office after a long history of being evaluated for problems such as anemia, fatigue, fever, and weight loss without explanation. Less often the onset of SLE is sudden and dramatic, with bleeding from the lungs, kidney problems, or multiple organ involvement. Again, it is important to remember that SLE is not the only disease that may cause these findings.

Once the diagnosis of SLE is suspected, proper evaluation begins with testing for ANA. As noted, if the ANA test is negative, it is extremely unlikely that the child has SLE. If the test for ANA is positive, further evaluation should include a complete blood count (CBC), chemistry panel, clotting studies, urinanalysis, and testing for Ro, La, Sm, RNP, and anti-DNA antibodies (see Chapter 22). Measurements of complement levels C3 and C4 should be performed. It is also useful to screen these children for thyroid function abnormalities, antithyroid antibodies, anticardiolipin antibodies, and rheumatoid factor. Sometimes after these tests it will be clear that a child has SLE. In other cases, there are several abnormalities but not enough to make a definite diagnosis of SLE.

The diagnosis of definite SLE requires that the child fulfill four of the eleven American College of Rheumatology criteria for the diagnosis of definite lupus. However, there are many children with SLE who initially fulfill fewer than four criteria. If children have several findings that suggest SLE but do not fulfill criteria for a definite diagnosis of SLE, they should be monitored carefully. It really does not matter whether they are said to have SLE, possible SLE, or probable SLE. The key to proper care for these children is to treat appropriately whatever problems they are having.

Children who have nonspecific symptoms and a positive ANA require routine follow-up to look for evidence of disease. Some physicians simply instruct the parents to bring the child back if more problems develop. I prefer to be proactive and periodically look for problems. This often allows me to begin therapy before the problems become more serious. It is well known that children with SLE may develop kidney disease and damage to other organs without initially complaining of pain or discomfort. It is important to detect these problems as early as possible and to minimize the damage to vital organs.

CLINICAL MANIFESTATIONS OF SLE

The patterns of disease involvement with SLE range from children with fever, rash, aches, and pains but no serious organ damage to children with no complaints of fever or rash who are found to have serious kidney or blood (hematologic) involvement on a routine screening test. Serious internal organ involvement most often takes the form of kidney involvement, but the brain, heart, lungs, and other internal organs also may be seriously affected.

Many children with SLE have a mild version that is easily treated by an experienced physician, but other children have more severe problems and have serious internal organ involvement. It is important to determine as far as possible which children have mild disease and which children have severe disease, though this cannot be done with absolute certainty. There are children who start out with mild disease and get worse over time. There are also some children who start out extremely ill, respond well to therapy, and do fine. The challenge for physicians and families caring for children with SLE is to find the proper balance between the side effects of medication and the risks of damage from the disease. When they can be recognized, children with severe disease should be treated aggressively before there is a lot of organ damage, not after.

Kidney Involvement in SLE

Kidney (renal) involvement is one of the most worrisome aspects of SLE. However, there are varying degrees of kidney involvement, from the very mild to the very severe. Approximately two-thirds of children with SLE will have at least mild kidney involvement at the time they are diagnosed. Most but not all children with significant kidney involvement have evident abnormalities on a urinalysis when they are first brought to the doctor.

In a child with obvious SLE, the physicians may elect to treat with corticosteroids, doing a kidney biopsy to determine the type of involvement only if the child does not respond to this treatment. Other physicians will biopsy every child with SLE, while some biopsy every child with SLE who has abnormal urine tests. There is no single correct answer. If your child has had a kidney biopsy, the pathologist will look at the tissue sample and report the type of kidney involvement according to the World Health Organization classification, with class I being a normal kidney and class V indicating the most severe damage. A class I or class II biopsy is not a cause for major concern. A Class III, IV, or V biopsy is worrisome. In addition to indicating the WHO classification, the biopsy report should contain immunofluorescence results, which indicate whether immunoglobulin or complement is being deposited in the kidney and in what parts.

Most physicians now believe that Class III involvement with strong evidence that immunoglobulin or complement is being deposited in the filtering areas of the kidney requires aggressive treatment as well, since these findings suggest the disease is likely to become worse over time.

A child with Class IV kidney involvement is at serious risk of kidney damage and even failure and must be treated appropriately. If you are told that your child has a class IV biopsy, you need to know the "activity" score, which measures inflammation in the kidney, and the "chronicity" score, which estimates the amount of scarring in the kidney. If the chronicity index is very high, it does not make sense to treat the child aggressively, as badly scarred kidneys are not going to recover. The key to a successful outcome is to catch the involvement early and prevent the chronicity index from going up over time. Class V biopsies indicate the serious kidney damage called membranous nephritis, which causes a whole host of problems. When enough of the kidneys' filtering system has failed, the kidneys are no longer effective and the child is in renal failure, which must be treated with dialysis and transplantation.

Intravenous cyclophosphamide is the only drug that has been shown to prevent the progression of kidney failure. The higher the class of biopsy, the less well it is likely to work, but we do not have anything that is clearly better. There is increasing evidence that rituximab can be beneficial as well. These drugs do have side effects, but they are far less problematic than long-term dialysis or the lifetime of immunosuppression required following kidney transplantation.

Brain and Nervous System Involvement in SLE

Seizures, strokes, and other serious abnormalities are possible but relatively infrequent consequences of SLE. Brain damage due to strokes is usually very dramatic. It can result in sudden inability to use a hand, leg, or whole side of the body. Sometimes the stroke may affect a speech center, making it impossible for the child to talk, or the balance centers, making the child unable to walk normally. Whenever there is a sudden change in the ability of a child with SLE to function normally, the brain should be carefully evaluated.

Subtle problems due to brain involvement are more common and vary from difficulty with fine motor skills and poor penmanship to suddenly worsening grades and severe depression. These stem from a combination of the physical effects of SLE, the effects of the medications needed to control it, and the child's reaction to having a serious chronic illness; it is difficult if not impossible to separate out these components.

A number of tests are used to evaluate a child with SLE who is showing neurologic abnormalities. An MRI will show structural changes in the brain. It will also show increased water content, which can occur with inflammation, bleeding, or other problems. A CAT scan will show structural problems and may also demonstrate bleeding, among other problems. When these tests are normal, some physicians will recommend a spinal tap to test the cerebrospinal fluid for the presence of sugar, protein, cells, or immunoglobulins. All of these may be abnormal if SLE is affecting the brain. They also may all be normal. The most important reason to look at the cerebrospinal fluid in this situation is to make sure there is no infection or other unsuspected problem. Nuclear isotope brain scans called SPECT scans are utilized by some medical centers to evaluate brain function but are generally considered unreliable in SLE.

Heart Involvement in SLE

Mild heart involvement is common in children with SLE but does not usually become significant. Pericarditis (involvement of the pericardium, the fibrous sac containing the heart) may cause chest pain that may worsen with deep breaths or changing position, such as leaning forward. Pericarditis can be detected easily with an echocardiogram. Children with chest pain must also be evaluated for pulmonary emboli (see "Lung Involvement in SLE," below). Minor thickening of the pericardium is often found in children with SLE who do not report chest pain, but if a child reports chest pain and there is thickening of the pericardium, an NSAID may help. Another common result of pericardial inflammation that can be seen on an echocardiogram is pericardial effusion, a painless increase in the amount of fluid around the heart. This fluid can ultimately interfere with the strength of the heartbeat and produce shortness of breath, swollen feet, and other signs of poor heart output (heart failure).

It is rare but possible for the heart muscle to become significantly inflamed in children with SLE. If myocarditis is present, there may be chest pain and there will be an increase in the blood level of creatine kinase (CK), an enzyme that is found in both heart muscle and other tissues; the laboratory can determine whether the CK is coming from the heart, other muscles, the brain, or elsewhere. Myocarditis may cause abnormalities in the heart rhythm that will show up on an electrocardiogram (EKG). It may also interfere with the ability of the heart to pump blood, producing symptoms of poor heart output.

Buildup of abnormal material on the surface of the heart valves is another common cause of problems in children with SLE. This is termed Libman-Sacks endocarditis. This is worrisome because the accumulated fibrous material may interfere with the proper opening and closing of the valve, forcing the heart to work harder and possibly pushing it into failure. These fibrous deposits also provide a place for bacteria to grow. Usually our bodies simply eliminate the harmful bacteria that occasionally find their way into our bloodstream, but if the bacteria start growing in these deposits, they may spread through the bloodstream to any part of the body. The bacteria may also worsen the heart valves' function and possibly cause a piece of the fibrous deposits to break off, potentially causing a stroke or other tissue damage or causing infection elsewhere in the body. To minimize these risks, children and adults with any type of heart valve involvement must take antibiotics before they go to the dentist; some doctors give antibiotics before dental visits to all the children they treat with serious SLE, even if they do not have definite heart valve involvement.

Heart valve involvement is usually detected by an echocardiogram. This will show how well the heart is beating, the motion of the valves, and any significant deposits around the valves. In some situations the physician may need to do a transesophageal echocardiogram (TE echo), which involves swallowing a transducer so that the physicians can look at the heart from another direction. It's hardly comfortable, but it does give a much better picture.

Treatment of heart involvement varies with the type and severity of the involvement. Mild pericarditis may be treated with NSAIDs. More severe pericarditis is often treated with corticosteroids. In rare cases, this does not work or the problem recurs frequently or is very severe. When that happens, it may be necessary for a surgeon to open up the pericardium to relieve the pressure on the heart. In general, this type of surgery has to be done only once and will permanently solve the problem.

The treatment of Libman-Sacks endocarditis is much more of a problem. If the fibrous deposits on the valves are small, the doctors may choose to leave them alone. If they are breaking off and causing problems, the child may have to be given blood thinners (anticoagulants). If they are infected, a long-term course of antibiotics is required. If too much damage has occurred, it may be necessary to do open-heart surgery and replace the valve. Fortunately, with modern aggressive therapy this problem is becoming rare.

Another problem for children with SLE is the development of arteriosclerosis, the hardening of the arteries that occurs normally as people get older. In its severe forms, it causes narrowing of the coronary arteries, which leads to heart attack. Chronic use of corticosteroids promotes the development of arteriosclerosis, so children who have received a lot of corticosteroids may develop arteriosclerosis in their teens or twenties. High cholesterol levels (which may occur in children with severe kidney damage) also promote arteriosclerosis. High blood pressure may be a consequence of corticosteroids and/or kidney disease. Inflammation in the blood vessels promotes high blood pressure and arteriosclerosis, too. Some children with SLE have all of these factors. As a result, a number of children with lupus who have been treated with moderate doses of corticosteroids for many years will have a heart attack in their twenties or thirties. This is one of the strongest arguments for using powerful immunosuppressive drugs early in SLE to bring it under control and minimize the amount of corticosteroids that the child takes over time.

Lung Involvement in SLE

Lung involvement in children with SLE may take several different forms. Most children with SLE never experience lung symptoms. However, weakening of the diaphragm (the muscle that moves the lungs) is a common problem in children with SLE. This makes it more difficult for children with SLE to take a really deep breath or to cough deeply. This poor air movement combined with medications that interfere with the immune response makes children with SLE more vulnerable to pneumonia. In children with SLE, pneumonia needs to be treated aggressively.

Some children with SLE are found to have areas of inflammation in the lungs that are diagnosed as fibrosis, a stiffening of the air sacs (alveoli) in the lungs. Small areas of fibrosis are not important and usually disappear with treatment of the SLE. Occasionally children develop more severe cases of fibrosis, which may interfere with the ability of the lungs to move air in and out. If this progresses over time, it can be quite serious. In rare cases, children with areas of lung involvement may form pockets of nonfunctional air cells, or "blebs." If an area of fibrosis or a bleb breaks, air can leak out of the lungs and into the chest cavity. This is called a pneumothorax. When this happens, the child will experience severe chest pain and difficulty breathing, and must be taken to the hospital by ambulance immediately. Fortunately, this problem is uncommon.

Blood clots (pulmonary emboli) may occur in the lungs of children with SLE. The symptoms in children are the sudden onset of chest pain and shortness of breath. Although children with clotting problems and anticardiolipin antibodies are at greater risk of developing pulmonary emboli (see "Hematologic Involvement in SLE," below), children without these findings may also have this problem. Any child with sudden onset of pain and shortness of breath or severe chest pain must be promptly evaluated. Blood clots may be diagnosed on the basis of X-rays, CAT scans, MRIs, or ventilation-perfusion (VQ) scans. Some newer tests such as D-dimer assays to detect blood clotting problems are also being evaluated. Children with blood clots will have to be treated with anticoagulants.

Some children with SLE develop serositis, an inflammation of the cells that line the inside of the chest or abdominal cavity (see "Gastrointestinal System Involvement in SLE," below). When this occurs in the chest, it causes pain and difficulty in breathing. The symptoms are very similar to those of pericarditis and the two can be reliably distinguished only with an echocardiogram. The symptoms may also mimic those of a pulmonary embolus.

Pulmonary hemorrhage, or bleeding in the lungs, is a very serious complication of SLE. It is the result of chronic irritation of the blood vessels in the lungs. For oxygen to be moved from the air breathed into the lungs to the blood vessels in the lungs, the blood vessels must be very close to the surface of the alveoli, or air sacs. If the blood vessels are very irritated by inflammation, they may begin leaking blood into the alveoli. This prevents the proper exchange of oxygen. Poor heart function will make this worse, because it results in increased blood pressure in the lungs (pulmonary hypertension), which leads to increased bleeding. If a child is coughing up blood, he or she should be taken to the physician immediately; often a small amount of blood is coming from irritation in the airway or from blood swallowed because of a cut in the nose or mouth, but it is best to make sure. If a child really is bleeding inside the lung, there is no time to waste, so if a child is getting short of breath and acting as if he or she is not getting enough oxygen, go to a hospital immediately.

Hematologic Involvement in SLE

Hematologic involvement refers to involvement of the blood-making system in the bone marrow or a problem in the mechanism of blood clotting. The most common hematologic involvement in SLE is anemia, or too few red blood cells. Whenever there is a problem with the number of a particular type of cell that comes from the bone marrow, physicians have to ask whether too few cells are being made or whether the cells are being used up too fast. In children with SLE, both answers may apply.

Red blood cell involvement is most often anemia of chronic disease. This comes from poor uptake and use of iron; as a result, too few red blood cells are being made. However, if a child is bleeding (from an ulcer, from the kidneys, from heavy menses, or many other sources), he or she will be anemic because the blood is being lost. Some children with SLE develop hemolytic anemia, a condition in which the body is destroying its own red blood cells because they have abnormal antibodies on their surface. Anemia of chronic disease results in a low hemoglobin and a low reticulocyte count. (Reticulocytes are newly made red cells.) Bleeding will result in a high reticulocyte count if the body has enough iron stores. If there is bleeding, the doctor should be able to find where it is occurring. Hemolytic anemia is suggested by finding low hemoglobin with a very high reticulocyte count without bleeding. It can be confirmed by special tests to detect antibodies on the red blood cells.

White blood cell involvement is most often leucopenia (having too few white blood cells). It may result from the cells being used up very quickly in trying to fight an infection. It can also be the result of the cells being destroyed because of anti-white-cell antibodies in the blood. Another possibility is that not enough white cells are being made in the bone marrow. This may be due to drugs, infections, or the SLE itself. Children with SLE often have normal white blood cell counts. High white cell counts can occur but need to be investigated as possible evidence of infection.

Severe leukopenia (under 1,000 white cells/mm^3) is worrisome because there may be too few of the cells needed to fight infection. If the level is too low, the doctor may wish to give drugs to stimulate white cell growth. Any child with a low white blood cell count and a fever should be promptly checked by the doctor for evidence of infection. Children who develop large scabs on their lips without having been injured may be getting an infection from the normal bacteria in the mouth. This is often a sign of a dangerously low white blood cell count.

Platelets are the third major type of blood cell made in the bone marrow. They are the sticky cells that float around in the blood and immediately adhere to any damaged surface to start formation of a clot and limit bleeding. If the number drops too low, the child will bruise easily. With very low numbers, the child may start to bruise without doing anything. If your child has SLE and is starting to bruise too easily, make sure the doctor knows. If you look inside your child's mouth with a flashlight and see bruises on the inside of the cheeks, next to the teeth, that may mean the platelet count is very low. Call the doctor and insist on being seen immediately.

Any hematologic abnormality that occurs in a child with SLE needs to be investigated. Corticosteroids treat most of them satisfactorily. If the problems are persistent or recurrent, there are other therapies. Surprisingly, cyclophosphamide has proven useful for these conditions, though it has to be given with great care and only by someone with appropriate experience. Rituximab has proven very effective for many children with low platelet counts.

Some children with SLE have inadequate clotting and bleed too much; girls with SLE are sometimes recognized because of excessive bleeding with their periods (menorrhagia). Children with SLE may make antibodies that interfere with the way the cells are supposed to stick together to form a clot. The antibodies that interfere with clotting in different children with SLE may be very different from each other. In addition, over time they may change slightly. This is important because while people with these antibodies sometimes bleed too much, sometimes they have the opposite problem and their blood clots too easily; occasionally a child will have both problems at the same time. Children with anticardiolipin (ACL) or antiphospholipid (APL) antibodies need to be monitored and their bodies prevented from making the antibodies. Corticosteroids can do this, and so can other immunosuppressive drugs. Early studies suggest that rituximab may be helpful.

There is a lot of controversy over what to do with children who have ACL or APL antibodies. If a child has had a clot, he or she has to be treated with anticoagulants. However, many children test positive for ACL or APL but have never had a problem. It might seem obvious to treat them with anticoagulants, but then if they get cut or fall they may bleed too much. It does not seem worth the risk for a child who has never had a problem. Some physicians feel it is best to just watch; others believe you should treat with a baby aspirin every day to try to decrease the risk. There is no certain answer. Children who have had problems with blood clots must be treated with anticoagulants (e.g., heparin and warfarin).

Gastrointestinal System Involvement in SLE

Irritation of the GI system occurs frequently in children with SLE. It may play a large role in the initial malaise that many children with SLE experience. The resulting pain and loss of appetite often lead to depression and weight loss. These are common problems in the period before diagnosis (note that this can happen in many other conditions as well). The most common GI complaint of children with SLE is nonspecific stomachache (abdominal pain). This can be located almost anywhere in the abdomen. It may be associated with eating, or it may not. Often the first thought of the family and physician is that it is the result of irritation from the medications the child is taking. If it persists, everyone becomes worried about ulcers, though children with SLE do not often get ulcers except when the disease is very severe and active.

The typical stomach irritation associated with medications is gastritis. If all the medicines are important, it is often better to treat the irritation with medicines to prevent acid secretion or coat the stomach (e.g., an H2 acid blocker or sucralfate). If these steps do not work, talk to your doctor about stopping the medicine if possible (steroids should never be discontinued abruptly, however; see Chapter 20) and see whether the pain goes away. If it does, restart the medicine. If the pain promptly comes back, that's a strong indication that the medicine is the cause. You and your doctor will then have to see whether there is an alternative medication that may be used.

Chronic abdominal pain in a child with SLE that is not resolved by changing medications needs to be carefully investigated. Some children have sensitive stomachs, but more serious problems can also begin with these complaints. One of the key aspects of SLE is inflammation of the blood vessels. If the blood vessels lining the intestines are inflamed, it may cause vague nonspecific pain. In some children this results in damage to the intestinal tract. This may take the form of pneumatosis cystoides intestinalis (gas-filled cysts in the wall of the bowel) or small areas of bowel where tissue has died because they do not receive enough blood. Both of these problems are difficult to diagnose on routine examination.

They are rare in children whose SLE is well controlled, but they must be looked for by an experienced physician in children whose complaints continue.

Another cause of chronic pain in children with SLE is serositis, inflammation of the lining of the lungs or abdomen (serosa). An inflamed serosa will respond by releasing inflammatory cells and inflammatory chemicals into the abdomen. In mild cases this causes diffuse pain. In severe cases the pain may be quite marked and associated with rebound tenderness (the child experiences pain when the abdomen is pressed but worse pain when the pressure is quickly released). Any child with this problem needs to be evaluated promptly by a physician, as it is an indication of serious irritation in the abdomen. There are many possible causes, including infections. If SLE is determined to be the cause, it may need to be better controlled with more corticosteroids or immunosuppressive drugs.

Irritation of the pancreas is another cause of chronic abdominal pain in children with SLE. When the pancreas is irritated, it will leak digestive enzymes that normally go into the intestine to help digest food. When they leak into the bloodstream or the abdomen they cause pain and discomfort, a condition called pancreatitis. The levels of these enzymes can be measured in the blood and will be elevated if the child has pancreatitis. Your doctor will have to be very careful in analyzing this; irritation of the pancreatic from SLE itself requires more medicine, but drug-caused irritation requires less.

Other organs in the GI tract that may be irritated are the liver and the gallbladder. Gallbladder disease is particularly common in children with hemolytic anemia. This is easily detected on abdominal ultrasound. Usually it can be followed conservatively, but if the gallbladder is very involved or has a lot of stones, it may need to be removed. Children with liver involvement often have an enlarged liver that can be felt on examination and may be tender. Elevation of the liver enzymes on the blood tests will confirm this (see Chapter 22).

The spleen is another organ in the abdomen that may also be enlarged in children with SLE. It is not really part of the GI tract; it is part of the immune system. An enlarged spleen may cause pain on the left side of the abdomen.

When children with SLE have abdominal pain, sometimes initial tests will be normal, but repeat testing a few weeks later will show problems. Children with continuing abdominal pain without adequate explanation may need blood tests, X-rays, abdominal ultrasound, and either an MRI or a CAT scan of the abdomen to look for explanations. Consultation with a gastroenterologist and endoscopy may be necessary.

CHILDREN WITH SLE AND JOINT PROBLEMS

Although the family may not be aware of it, arthritis is often present when a child with SLE first comes to the doctor. It is usually very responsive to treatment with steroids or NSAIDs. As a result, arthritis is rarely a significant long-term problem. The exception is an unusual condition termed Jaccoud's arthropathy, a painless swelling, primarily in the fingers and wrists, that develops slowly during the course of SLE. It does not usually cause damage to the bones, but it may be painful and interfere with use of the hands. The explanation for this problem is unclear. Unfortunately, it does not respond well to medication.

Other bone and joint problems may develop during the treatment of children with SLE. The most common serious problem is avascular necrosis of bone. Although the mechanism by which this occurs is not fully understood, the death of bone cells and the resultant crumbling appears to be the result of decreased blood flow to the ends of the bones. While it occurs under a number of circumstances, it is most common in children with SLE who are being treated with corticosteroids. The problem often begins with vague complaints of pain in the involved bone without any findings on examination.

Early in the development of avascular necrosis, X-rays will be normal. Sometimes avascular necrosis is suspected on bone scans because there is decreased uptake of the radionuclide by the involved bone (see Chapter 22). MRI is the most sensitive test for this condition and will detect it very early. Sometimes children with a suggestion of avascular necrosis on MRI go on to recover. We do not know whether this means that the MRI was a false reading or whether early avascular necrosis is able to be reversed. However, if a child has definite avascular necrosis on MRI, it does not go away.

Unfortunately, the normal course of avascular necrosis is for the bone to crumble slowly under the continued stress of bearing weight. If this happens, it will be necessary for the joint to be replaced (see Chapter 23). In children with SLE, the hip is the joint most commonly affected, but shoulders, elbows, knees, ankles, and other joints all may be involved. The identical problem may occur in children with juvenile arthritis who have been treated with corticosteroids. There is no safe dose of corticosteroids with regard to this problem. Avascular necrosis has occurred in children who never got any corticosteroids, but the more corticosteroids the child takes and the longer he or she takes them, the greater the risk. Children taking any significant amount of corticosteroids for more six months have a steadily increasing risk of developing avascular necrosis. In addition, a child who has had avascular necrosis in one joint is at greater risk of developing it in another joint. Reducing the risk of avascular necrosis is one of the reasons physicians try so hard to minimize the dose of corticosteroids for children with SLE.

LABORATORY TESTING AND TYPICAL PATTERNS OF DISEASE IN CHILDREN WITH SLE

SLE is an enormously variable illness. Different patterns of abnormalities may help to distinguish children with severe disease from others with milder cases, helping to ensure they get appropriate treatment before significant damage occurs.

Virtually all of the children with SLE are ANA-positive. However, many children test positive for ANA but do not have SLE. Physicians soon recognized that there were different patterns of ANA as seen under the microscope (see Chapter 22 for more on this). Although a child with any ANA pattern could have problems, children with a "rim pattern" were much more likely to be very sick.

Further study led to the recognition that children with rim-pattern ANA often have antibodies to double-stranded DNA. Anti-dsDNA antibodies tend to be associated with more severe SLE and are only infrequently found in children who do not have SLE. However, a child may be very sick with SLE and not have antibodies to dsDNA. At one time these antibodies were thought to correlate with a greater frequency of renal disease, but this is now in doubt.

Further evaluation of patients with SLE led to the discovery of the extractable nuclear antigens Ro, La, Sm, and RNP (see Chapter 22). A lot of time and effort have gone into determining the importance of antibodies to these antigens. They do seem to be associated with different patterns of disease, but again there is not enough certainty to make definitive predictions. The clearest associations are with Ro and Sm. Often Ro antibodies are found in children with more rash, greater than average complaints of arthritis, and relatively less kidney disease. A high titer of Ro, high RNP, and low or absent Sm have been described as typical of mixed connective tissue disease (MCTD; see Chapter 10). Over the years a variety of studies have suggested that adults with SLE who are Ro-positive have milder disease, but it is a generalization that does not always hold true. Ro antibodies are also associated with neonatal SLE and congenital heart block, discussed at the end of this chapter.

The other antibody that seems to be important is Sm. This antibody is not found in everyone with SLE. If it is present, it is associated with a greater frequency of severe disease. However, just as the association of Ro with mild disease is only approximate, so is the association of Sm with severe disease. Indeed, some children have antibodies to both Ro and Sm. Do not get too concerned about which antibodies your child does or does not have, as children with problematic antibodies may do well and others with protective antibodies may get in big trouble. Make sure you have a good doctor and that the doctor is taking good care of your child's problems.

The key laboratory findings in evaluating a child with SLE are generally similar to those of children with other chronic illnesses. If a child is doing well, he or she should have a good hemoglobin level, a normal erythrocyte sedimentation rate, and a normal urinanalysis (though neurologic problems may still occur). ANA levels and anti-dsDNA levels rise and fall in children with SLE without a reliable association with disease activity. Any one test changing does not mean too much, but if they all start going the wrong way, be sure to pay attention.

The complement system, a group of proteins found in the blood, plays an important role in attacking infectious agents. In the course of doing their job, the different components of the complement system are used up. Although the body is constantly making more, a drop in the level of the complement components in the blood suggests very active usage. This is true in children with SLE as well. We know that much of the damage in SLE is brought about by the activation of complement following the deposition of immune complexes in the tissues. As a general rule, lower complement levels in the blood suggest a greater amount of ongoing damage. This is an imperfect system because doctors recognize that the levels in the blood are determined as much by how fast more is being made as by how fast it is being used up. There are very sophisticated tests to measure what are called complement breakdown products, but these tests are not routinely done. All the laboratory findings in children with SLE are individual pieces of the puzzle: some tell the physician how the organs are functioning right now, and others give some idea of the future course of the disease (though nothing is a perfect predictor).

DRUG-INDUCED SLE

Drug-induced SLE refers to the development of a positive ANA and SLE-like symptoms in association with certain drugs. Among the drugs that can do this are commonly used medications such as tetracyclines (including doxycycline, used in the treatment of teenagers with acne), certain of the drugs used to treat children with seizures, and some antibiotics (including isoniazid, used to treat tuberculosis). For some drugs, the association with drug-induced SLE is well known, but for many others it is only suspected. The fact that a medication has been associated with drug-induced SLE does not mean that it should not be used, for this is a rare complication. However, when evaluating a child with the new onset of SLE-like symptoms, these drugs should always be considered as a possible cause.

Children with drug-induced SLE can be significantly ill with fever, rash, and inflammation around the lungs or in the abdomen. However, a key to the diagnosis of drug-induced SLE is that it all goes away quickly if the drug is discontinued. If symptoms of SLE begin after a child has started on a drug but do not go away when the drug is stopped, it is not drug-induced SLE, even if it is a medication that is known to cause drug-induced SLE.

I am often asked whether a child who has SLE can use a drug that is known to cause drug-induced SLE. Some of the most important drugs for treating hypertension (a common SLE complication) in the past were also known to cause drug-induced SLE, but there is no evidence they caused additional problems in children with SLE. Still, it is important to pay attention to the possibility of side effects arising over time.

COMPLICATIONS OF SLE

Complications of SLE in childhood may be complications of the disease, of the therapy, or of both. It is very important to understand that half of the children diagnosed with SLE in the 1950s (before the routine use of corticosteroids) died within two years. While diagnosis and treatment have improved and the picture is much brighter today, it remains true that untreated SLE may be a rapidly fatal disease. While treatment certainly has possible side effects, those must be balanced with the risk of inadequate treatment.

Severe complications of SLE, such as pulmonary hemorrhage, renal failure, and strokes, have all become less frequent with proper therapy. Children with active SLE often have poorly functioning white blood cells and reduced levels of complement. Since these are key elements in the defense against infection, children with active SLE are more vulnerable to infection than normal children.

Another problem that leads to an increased frequency of infections is that children with active SLE often have a spleen that is not functioning well. Removing bacteria and other infectious agents from the blood is a major function of this organ. Children who do not have a spleen (because of surgical removal due to injury or other reasons) are well known to have more frequent pneumococcal infections. Systemic pneumococcal infections and pneumococcal pneumonia also occur more often in children with SLE. Meningococcal meningitis is another infection that occurs more often than expected in children with SLE. One important key to recognizing that the spleen is not functioning well in a child with SLE is the presence of Howell-Jolly bodies (leftover nuclear material in red blood cells) on the complete blood count. A normally functioning spleen removes this material. (Note that someone who has had the spleen removed will always have Howell-Jolly bodies and will always be at increased risk of infection, but the physician should know this.)

Parents are the most important line of defense against severe infection in children with SLE. You cannot lock your children in the closet to prevent them from ever being exposed to infections. You have to let them lead normal lives. However, do not let your child with SLE visit someone you know is sick. More important, if your child looks sick to you, insist that the doctor see him or her. A normal child who looks sick in the evening might safely wait until morning. In a child with active SLE, the normal defenses are not working and it may not be safe to wait until morning. Too, the medications used to treat SLE decrease the child's ability to fight infection. Any child on a significant dose of corticosteroids or any amount of immunosuppressive drugs such as methotrexate, cyclophosphamide, or azathioprine is at increased risk of infection.

In some cases a child with SLE will be brought to the hospital looking extremely ill and it is not clear whether the problem is an infection or a flare-up of the SLE. For an infection one would use an antibiotic, but for a flare-up of the SLE more corticosteroids are the answer. More corticosteroids, however, might make an infection worse. The best answer is to give both antibiotics and corticosteroids in this situation. Often the infection makes the SLE flare up, and this interferes with the ability of the white cells to fight infection. Other times the child came down with an infection because the SLE was flaring and again the white cells weren't able to fight infection. In either situation, using both corticosteroids and antibiotics is appropriate.

TREATMENT OF SLE

Corticosteroids have been a key element in the treatment of SLE since their discovery in the 1950s. They are effective in treating and preventing many of the complications of untreated SLE. However, they increase the incidence of infection, interfere with growth, weaken bones, cause stretch marks, promote diabetes, and hasten arteriosclerosis and heart disease (see Chapter 20).

For the one-third of children with mild disease (rash, malaise, and arthritis but no evidence of significant renal or other internal organ involvement), initial therapy should be with a low dose of corticosteroids. Often this is combined with an NSAID to provide some additional symptomatic relief. (There are, however, reports of NSAIDs causing unusual reactions such as aseptic meningitis in SLE patients.) Over the longer term the antimalarial drug hydroxychloroquine (see Chapter 20) has been shown to be very beneficial for this group. The child should feel better and any laboratory abnormalities should improve over a period of four to six weeks. As soon as it is clear that this has happened, the physician should try to begin slowly reducing the corticosteroids.

Unfortunately, the remaining two-thirds of children with SLE may face a recurrent need to raise the corticosteroid dosage to a more significant level. This brings with it an increased risk of corticosteroid-related toxicity. Surprisingly, this is a greater problem for children with moderate disease than for the children with severe disease (that is, those with internal organ involvement). Children with severe disease are usually rapidly recognized and advanced to more aggressive immunosuppressive therapy, which normally allows a dramatic reduction in the dosage of corticosteroids. As a result, corticosteroid-related complications are often less frequent in this group. After recognizing this, many physicians have begun to advocate advancing children with more difficult moderate SLE to immunosuppressive therapy early in their disease course in order to minimize corticosteroid-related toxicity. Though the immunosuppressants too can have significant side effects, these are very rare when given by an experienced practitioner. The key to proper treatment of SLE involves balancing the risks of the disease against the risks of the treatment.

In severe flares of SLE, an initial high dose of corticosteroid may be needed to control disease manifestations. In certain situations such as severe renal disease, it is often advisable to combine cyclophosphamide with the corticosteroids until the disease comes under better control. However, this is not a long-term solution because of the side effects of steroids. After the child improves, I recommend a gradual reduction in the corticosteroid dosage rather than a sudden drop-off. Even when physicians go very slowly, however, it is impossible to predict how much the corticosteroid dosage can be decreased before there is new evidence of disease activity. If it is possible to reduce the corticosteroids to 0.2 mg/kg/day of prednisone or its equivalent or less without recurrent disease, the child should be carefully followed on this low dose. Many parents are anxious to have their child discontinue steroids, but completely stopping corticosteroids is rarely advisable for children with SLE.

Cyclosporine is a strong immunosuppressive drug that often interferes with kidney function (see Chapter 20). It is known to cause kidney problems, and this has kept most physicians from using it for the treatment of SLE. However, there are occasional reports of its successful use. It seems especially useful to prevent progression of kidney disease in children with signs of serious kidney problems.

Children who do not have internal organ involvement but develop more symptoms when the dose of corticosteroids is reduced are a difficult problem. Hydroxychloroquine often helps to bring the disease under adequate control. Some physicians have tried using low-dose methotrexate in this group, but the results are highly variable. Without evidence of internal organ involvement physicians are hesitant to recommend more aggressive therapy, but that may leave a child on too high a dose of corticosteroids for too long. In my own experience, children in this group who do not tolerate appropriate reduction of their corticosteroids usually progress to have evidence of internal organ involvement over time. It is important for physicians to monitor them carefully. Frequently the first signs of internal organ involvement are small changes in the urinalysis.

A variety of "steroid-sparing" regimens have been recommended for children with SLE who need aggressive therapy. Mycophenolate mofetil is one of the most commonly recommended immunosuppressive medications at present (see Chapter 22), while other children do better on low-dose methotrexate or azathioprine. None of them is always effective. I often use two courses of therapy with rituximab and cyclophosphamide in these children with good results (each course consists of two treatments separated by two weeks and the courses are separated by six months).

New biologic agents and other experimental therapies are being tested in SLE. Some centers are also testing the use of autologous bone marrow transplants or very high doses of cyclophosphamide that completely suppress the immune system. At present their use is restricted to specialized centers and they are being used only for children who have failed normal therapy.

There is no perfect answer for children with SLE at the present time. Years of experience and seeing what happens to children over time have made me very aggressive in trying to prevent the side effects of long-term corticosteroid usage. I have found that children who have disease in any internal organ system that is not well controlled by an acceptable dose of corticosteroids do best if aggressively treated. Not every physician agrees, however, and it is the parents who must always make the final decision.

PROGNOSIS FOR CHILDREN WITH SLE

Despite the foregoing information about how the most difficult cases are treated, you should know that with early and aggressive treatment the vast majority of children do just fine. Some children do die from SLE, but the survival rate at five years is above 90 percent in every experienced center, and in some centers it is much higher. Of course, thinking just in terms of five-year survival is certainly not good enough for a fourteen-, fifteen-, or sixteen-year-old child. The main reason for advocating early aggressive therapy is that we want to achieve excellent forty-, fifty-, and sixty-year survival. We have no proof yet; someone will have to follow these children for fifty years into the future to prove that we've done the right thing. But we cannot keep doing what we know does not work while we wait forty or fifty years to get proof of the right long-term answers. Research is ongoing, and I will be very disappointed if we don't have completely different answers about how to best treat children with SLE long before fifty years from now.

Because most children with SLE in fact do quite well, sometimes a difficult issue for the families of children with SLE is sun exposure. Children with SLE want to play outside and go to the beach like other kids. However, it is well documented that the sun damages superficial skin cells and causes cell death. In normal individuals the body disposes of these damaged cells with minimal difficulty. In patients with SLE, however, this process is defective and the damaged cells remain in the skin for a prolonged period, likely stimulating the immune system to produce ANA and other antibodies that drive SLE. As a result, significant sun exposure (or exposure to UV rays in a tanning salon) may lead to a severe flare-up of the underlying SLE. It is essential that children with SLE wear appropriate sun block and avoid significant exposure to ultraviolet radiation.

ANTI-RO ANTIBODIES AND NEONATAL SLE

It was a surprising finding when it was recognized that babies born with a problem called complete congenital heart block (in which there is interference with the transmission of the electrical signals that regulate the normal pumping motion of the heart) are often had mothers with SLE. Most mothers with SLE have healthy babies, and conversely, most babies with congenital heart block have healthy mothers. But when doctors began testing them, it was found that almost all of the normal, healthy mothers who gave birth to children with congenital heart block tested positive for antibodies to Ro. A few of these mothers had unrecognized SLE when examined carefully, and some of these mothers (but so far not most) have gone on to develop SLE years later.

At first doctors were very worried that Ro-positive women would be at high risk of having children with congenital heart block. This seems not to be the case. Most Ro-positive mothers have normal children. Even Ro-positive mothers who have had one child with heart block most often have normal children the next time. If a woman who is known to be Ro-positive becomes pregnant, she should be monitored carefully.

Evidence of congenital heart block can be detected before birth, and experienced doctors should be standing by to take care of the children when they are born. Most often congenital heart block is not life-threatening and can be treated with a pacemaker when the child is old enough to need it. Rarely, children with heart block are extremely sick and may not survive. The problem is sufficiently uncommon that we encourage women with SLE and antibodies to Ro to go ahead and have children when they are ready, but with careful monitoring during pregnancy.

Other complications that may occur in children of mothers with SLE include low levels of platelets, white cells, or red cells. These are thought to be the result of antibodies that have been passed from the mother to the child. These antibodies are usually cleared out of the child's system in a few days, and the problems are rarely severe. Other children of mothers with SLE may develop a rash when they are first exposed to the light, or develop mild inflammation of the liver. These are all well-recognized problems that normally resolve after a few days to a few weeks. Serious complications in the children of mothers with SLE are infrequent.

As previously noted, genetics plays a role in the development of SLE. However, the risk of a mother passing SLE on to her child is very small. Precise numbers are uncertain, but one in fifty is the best estimate. Thus, the child of a mother with SLE is more likely to get the disease than a random child, but it is far from a certain thing. If you are a woman with SLE considering whether or not to have children, the major concern is your health, not the risk of the child having SLE. Women with SLE should discuss the subject with their doctor and be evaluated for any risk factors such as antibodies to Ro or anticardiolipin antibodies so that appropriate steps can be taken to minimize problems.

10

Mixed Connective Tissue Disease

Children with mixed connective tissue disease (MCTD) are ANA-positive like children with SLE, but typically have high titers of antibodies to RNP as well. The precise relationship of MCTD to SLE and the other rheumatic diseases remains unclear. Symptoms of MCTD may also be characteristic of dermatomyositis and scleroderma. Obviously, these diseases are somehow interrelated, but there is no clear explanation yet. Although MCTD was originally described as a subtype of SLE, it is probably more closely related to scleroderma and dermatomyositis.

Children with MCTD typically are brought to the doctor because of cold, blue hands (Raynaud's phenomenon) and joint pains. They often have elevated muscle enzymes and rashes over the outer surfaces of their knees and elbows. Often they have a mild to moderate amount of arthritis, but they may not have been complaining about it. Children with MCTD usually do not have serious kidney involvement, but they may have some and it may become serious.

DIFFERENTIAL DIAGNOSIS OF MCTD AND LABORATORY FINDINGS

As noted, the clinical manifestations of MCTD overlap with dermatomyositis, SLE, JA, and early scleroderma. Consequently, physicians must rely more heavily on laboratory findings to confirm this diagnosis. The source of much of the confusion in diagnosing MCTD results from the unclear nature of the disease itself. Indeed, it is quite possible that we will ultimately realize that at least two different diseases have been grouped together as MCTD.

A high-titer speckled-pattern ANA is characteristic of MCTD. When the ANA subtypes are checked, children with MCTD are usually Ro-positive, RNP-positive, and Sm-negative (some have low-titer Sm). Because these children are often RF-positive, they may be referred for juvenile arthritis. Another finding is that these children may have very marked elevation of their quantitative immunoglobulins, especially IgG (see Chapter 22). What differentiates MCTD from SLE are the speckled pattern of the ANA, a positive test for rheumatoid factor, and usually normal serum complement levels. Antibodies to double-stranded DNA are sometimes found in children with MCTD.

As previously mentioned, children with MCTD often have many findings that are also seen in dermatomyositis and scleroderma. In more severe cases, children with MCTD often have Gottren's papules (sores over the knuckles) and nail fold capillary abnormalities. Although children with MCTD have elevated muscle enzymes and rash, they do not tend to evolve into dermatomyositis. However, MCTD may develop into scleroderma over a period of years. The presence of antibodies to Scl-70, or anticentromere antibodies, strongly suggests the diagnosis of scleroderma. These antibodies may not be present initially but may appear years later.

COMPLICATIONS OF MCTD

The complications of MCTD are highly dependent on the evolution of the disease. The arthritis, rash, malaise, and Raynaud's phenomenon are usually easily treated with NSAIDs, low-dose prednisone, a calcium-channel blocker for the Raynaud's, and hydroxychloroquine. Inadequately treated children may have recurrent problems with Raynaud's and may have distal fingertip ulcers and problems with blood supply to parts of the digits in the cold. Physicians must emphasize to families the importance of treating the Raynaud's and seeking care if a digit does not warm up appropriately with return to a warm environment. The elevated muscle enzymes and the markedly elevated IgG level will usually respond to a moderate or low dose of prednisone.

Children with fever and distress should be presumed to have poor spleen function and should be hospitalized and put on intravenous antibiotics until it is certain that they do not have an infection. If the laboratory reports Howell-Jolly bodies on the peripheral smear, this is evidence that the spleen is not functioning properly and there is an increased risk of infection. Some children with MCTD have poor blood circulation in their hands and feet. If the circulation to a finger or toe has stopped and it is numb and discolored, this is a reason for immediate hospitalization. In most cases a numb and discolored finger or toe responds to intravenous bolus methylprednisolone. A variety of regimens may be considered if this is not effective in restoring circulation.

Some children with MCTD will develop obvious scleroderma over time. Other children do not develop the typical skin changes of scleroderma but may develop shortness of breath and pulmonary function abnormalities. Pulmonary fibrosis (stiffening of the air sacs in the lungs) may occur, and I have seen children who developed a pneumothorax (leakage of air into the chest cavity) as a result. In other children, pulmonary fibrosis may result in pulmonary hypertension with resultant cardiac problems and an increased risk of infection.

Sudden overwhelming infection remains the most commonly reported cause of death for children with MCTD. This may be related to a high frequency of problems with the spleen, as discussed for children with SLE. Parents of children with MCTD should be prompt in seeking medical care at the first suspicion of a serious infection. Whenever possible, children with MCTD should receive vaccination against pneumococcal infections.

TREATMENT OF MCTD

The standard treatment for MCTD is a low dose of corticosteroids combined with hydroxychloroquine and an NSAID for relief of the arthritis. The corticosteroid dosage should be adjusted as necessary to correct the elevated IgG level, erythrocyte sedimentation rate, anemia, and clinical symptoms. Significant Raynaud's syndrome should be treated with an appropriate calcium-channel blocker. Although stronger agents are available if these do not provide relief, most children with MCTD will do well on this combination.

For some children with MCTD, it is not possible to reduce the corticosteroid dosage to a satisfactory level. Methotrexate seems to be an effective steroid-sparing agent for these children. Most often it is necessary to treat them with higher doses of methotrexate, as are used in dermatomyositis and scleroderma (i.e., up to 1 mg/kg/week, 50 mg maximum). The key to successful treatment of MCTD is early recognition of the children who are at high risk for progressive disease. Children in this group who are treated aggressively generally do well.

Stronger immunosuppressive agents rarely are necessary for the treatment of children with MCTD unless the condition is evolving toward scleroderma. For children who do not respond to or tolerate methotrexate, azathioprine or mycophenolate mofetil may be considered. In the small subset of children who develop kidney damage, treatment with intravenous cyclophosphamide may be necessary and is often helpful. Children who progress to scleroderma are difficult to treat and should be treated as appropriate for that condition (see Chapter 13).

PROGNOSIS FOR CHILDREN WITH MCTD

The long-term prognosis depends on the evolution of the disease. Most children do well with the treatment I have described. In many the disease seems to resolve slowly over time and the children are eventually able to discontinue all medications. However, children who develop significant lung involvement or other evidence of progression toward scleroderma need to be treated aggressively; even so, the prognosis is guarded, as it is for all children with scleroderma.

11

Sjögren's Syndrome

The combination of dry eyes and dry mouth that is characteristic of Sjögren's syndrome may be the result of inflammation of the glands that produce tears and saliva. Children with Sjögren's syndrome are often sent to the rheumatologist by a dentist who has noted that they have unusually severe cavities or by an ophthalmologist who has noted that their complaints of eye discomfort are due to chronically dry eyes and poor tear production. Most of these children are ANA-positive, and the majority test positive for antibodies to Ro (see below). Other children with Sjögren's syndrome are sent to the rheumatologist because of Raynaud's syndrome and a positive ANA or rheumatoid factor.

When they are evaluated, some of the children with Sjögren's syndrome clearly have SLE; these children are said to have secondary Sjögren's syndrome. Sjögren's syndrome is also a known complication of rheumatoid arthritis in adults, but it rarely occurs in children with juvenile arthritis. I have seen children with sarcoidosis who had Sjögren's syndrome and arthritis. Children who have dry eyes and dry mouth but lack other findings suggestive of connective tissue disease have primary Sjögren's syndrome. However, over time some children with what was thought to be primary Sjögren's syndrome ultimately develop more findings and are diagnosed with SLE. The only way to deal with this is to treat the Sjögren's appropriately (usually with hydroxychloroquine and low-dose steroids) and to monitor them carefully.

One source of confusion in caring for children with Sjögren's syndrome is the involvement of the acinar glands. The acinar glands include not only the parotid and submandibular glands, which produce saliva, but also the pancreas. All the acinar glands are part of the digestive process. The parotid and submandibular glands produce amylase just as the pancreas does, and if they are inflamed, the level of amylase in the blood will be elevated. Doctors often measure the amylase level if they suspect pancreatitis (see Chapter 22). However, in children with Sjögren's syndrome, an elevated amylase level may reflect inflammation of the parotid gland and not pancreatitis. Sometimes children with

Sjögren's do have simultaneous inflammation in the pancreas and the parotid glands, so a careful evaluation is important.

Some children who develop recurrent swelling of the parotid glands are diagnosed with recurrent epidemic parotitis. This used to be common before everyone was immunized against mumps (mumps virus infection often causes swelling of the parotid glands). However, in reality, many of these children have Sjögren's syndrome.

Children with Sjögren's syndrome may also be referred because they have developed arthritis. For this reason, I always ask questions about whether a child with arthritis has sores in the mouth or difficulty swallowing.

Kidney involvement with Sjögren's syndrome may take the form of blood or protein in the urine. There is also an association with a condition called renal tubular acidosis, in which the kidney loses its ability to regulate the amount of acid in the urine, affecting the body's acid/base balance. Children with this condition should be under the care of an experienced nephrologist.

COMPLICATIONS OF SJÖGREN'S SYNDROME

The most common complications of Sjögren's syndrome are a direct result of the dry eyes. Dry eyes are easily scratched, and the scratches (corneal abrasions) are both painful and ultimately damaging to the lens of the eye. These children need frequent monitoring by an ophthalmologist. The dry mouth results in a very high frequency of cavities, as saliva normally helps wash away the bacteria responsible for tooth decay. These complications can become quite serious, and it is important to make sure children use artificial tears and artificial saliva if they need them. Special toothpastes and medicines to increase saliva production also help.

Most of the other complications of Sjögren's syndrome respond well to treatment. The kidney involvement usually is responsive to appropriate treatment by nephrologists. Sometimes children with Sjögren's syndrome develop abdominal pain and a rash over the fronts of their legs. If they did not have the other findings, this would be considered Henoch-Schoenlein purpura. It is thought to result from the deposit of large immune complexes in the skin and intestines. Children with this complication may also develop a flare of their arthritis and other problems and should be evaluated carefully.

TREATMENT OF SJÖGREN'S SYNDROME

Artificial tears and artificial saliva are very important parts of the treatment of children with Sjögren's syndrome. Some teenagers are reluctant to use them at school for fear of seeming different. However, the dry eyes and dry mouth can do so much damage that it is very important to encourage routine use of artificial tears and saliva even at school.

Hydroxychloroquine is often helpful in slowing the progression of the disease. Corticosteroids are useful if the symptoms are more severe or progress despite the use of hydroxychloroquine. In severe cases methotrexate or another immunosuppressive agent may be necessary. Rituximab has shown promise in very severe adult cases and may be used in children with Sjögren's syndrome as well.

Children who develop ocular, dental, or renal problems need to be treated appropriately for these problems, which in most cases are not difficult to manage. There is an association between Sjögren's syndrome and lymphomas and Waldenstrom's macroglobulinemia (a rare chronic cancer of the plasma cells) in adults, but this is not generally true in childhood. Most children with primary Sjögren's syndrome do well.

PROGNOSIS FOR CHILDREN WITH
SJÖGREN'S SYNDROME

The long-term prognosis for children with primary Sjögren's syndrome is unclear. Some children develop other rheumatic diseases over time. In that case, the underlying rheumatic disease determines the prognosis. Failure to attend properly to recurrent ocular or dental problems may have significant consequences. Serious complications related to kidney disease and vasculitis are infrequent. Because Sjögren's syndrome is rare in childhood, there are no good reports describing the extended follow-up of children with this diagnosis.

12

Raynaud's Phenomenon

Maurice Raynaud (1834–1881) was a French medical student who noted color changes in the hands of some women while standing outside in the cold waiting for the streetcar during the winter in Paris. **Raynaud's phenomenon** refers to the typical hand changes he described. **Raynaud's disease** (primary Raynaud's) refers to the typical hand changes occurring in the absence of any other rheumatic disease. **Raynaud's syndrome** (secondary Raynaud's) refers to the typical changes occurring in the setting of an underlying rheumatic disease.

Many people experience cold hands whenever it is cool outside. This is not Raynaud's phenomenon. Raynaud's phenomenon results from spasm of the blood vessels in response to a stressor such as exposure to the cold or embarrassment. Many of my patients with significant Raynaud's syndrome describe their worst problems as occurring in the summer when they walk into air-conditioned buildings from the heat outside. The fundamental abnormality is the hyperreactivity of the blood vessels. Raynaud's may be the result of being thin (it is common for tall, thin women to have Raynaud's phenomenon) or of the blood vessels being sensitized by immune complexes or by inflammatory mediators (see Chapter 22) because the individual has an underlying rheumatic disease.

For a diagnosis of Raynaud's phenomenon, there must be a three-phase color change. Initially, the tips of one or more fingers turn white as the blood flow is cut off by spasm of the blood vessels. Once the spasm passes, there is increased reactive blood flow and the fingers turn red, then slowly go back to their normal state of bluish discoloration, with sluggish blood flow. Cold red hands or cold blue hands without the spasmodic white phase do not constitute Raynaud's phenomenon.

The importance of Raynaud's phenomenon lies in its association with a variety of rheumatic diseases. While Raynaud's is common in thin young women, it is often the first manifestation noticed in children with progressive systemic sclerosis (see Chapter 13). Raynaud's is also found frequently in children with other vasculitic diseases, such as lupus, dermatomyositis, and anticardiolipin antibody syndrome. It may occur in children with many other rheumatic conditions.

Since most young women with Raynaud's phenomenon are healthy, it is important to recognize children in whom Raynaud's is a warning of an underlying condition. Every child with Raynaud's should have routine testing done, but boys with Raynaud's are at greater risk of underlying disease than girls, and children less than twelve years of age are at greater risk than older children. Tall, thin girls with a family history of Raynaud's disease tend to have fewer problems with underlying disease than those without a family history. Long-lasting episodes of Raynaud's, a high frequency of episodes, shortness of breath, chest pain when the Raynaud's occurs, and morning stiffness (particularly in the fingers) all increase the probability that an underlying disease is present. When examining the child, the physician should look carefully for nail fold capillary abnormalities (see Fig. 12-1) or distal fingertip pitting (see below). Either of these findings substantially increases the probability of an underlying disease being present.

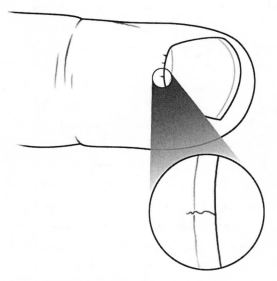

FIG 12-1 *Dilated nail fold capillaries may be easy to see with a small magnifying glass.*

Many physicians are concerned that they lack the proper equipment for nail fold capillary microscopy, but this can be easily done with an otoscope (the small handheld magnifier used for looking in ears). In a normal individual, the nail fold capillaries cannot be seen, even with an otoscope. If red streaks are seen in the nail folds, it suggests the presence of nail fold capillary abnormalities and the child should be referred for further evaluation. All ten fingers should be examined, as the presence of the abnormality on any finger is significant.

Distal fingertip pitting is another important finding that is also easily detected on routine examination. These pits are little areas where the blood supply has been cut off and the skin and underlying tissues have atrophied. As a result, the areas often feel callused to the examiner. The child will describe decreased feeling in the fingertips, as one would expect from calluses. If you look carefully, you may be able to see the areas of thickened skin, often with little central depressions or scars. However, it is easiest to screen for these by feeling the tips of the fingers. The areas that are scarred are harder than normal skin and feel like little bumps.

LABORATORY TESTING OF A CHILD WITH RAYNAUD'S

Laboratory evaluation of a child with Raynaud's should include a complete blood count, erythrocyte sedimentation rate, antinuclear antibody, rheumatoid factor, anticardiolipin antibodies, clotting studies, and thyroid function tests. If there are no suggestive findings on history or physical examination and all of these tests are normal, there is little likelihood of an underlying rheumatic disease. However, the presence of a positive ANA, positive RF, anticardiolipin antibodies, or an elevated ESR should all prompt more complete investigation, as should any suggestive findings on history or physical examination.

COMPLICATIONS OF RAYNAUD'S

If a child is known to have an underlying rheumatic disease, the presence of Raynaud's phenomenon does not necessarily indicate more serious disease. However, there are several complications related to Raynaud's that must be considered. In more severe cases, children with Raynaud's may have problems not only in their fingers but also in their toes, earlobes, and tip of the nose. All of these areas should be protected if the child is to be subjected to significant cold exposure.

It is also important to recognize that children with Raynaud's phenomenon may have increased reactivity in other blood vessels. This is a rare complication, but I have cared for children with scleroderma who had chest pain and cardiac abnormalities because their coronary arteries constricted whenever their fingers blanched because of Raynaud's phenomenon. If the internal organs are being deprived of blood flow, the Raynaud's must be treated aggressively to prevent damage to these organs.

Any child who has distal fingertip pitting or a history of severe Raynaud's should not be unnecessarily exposed to cold stress, as gangrene with loss of parts of fingers or toes can occur. Whenever a child has prolonged loss of circulation to a finger or toe, he or she should be taken to the emergency room. I tell my patients that if a finger is white and numb for more than ten minutes, they should be inside making every effort to warm it up. If it is not clearly back to normal after half an hour, they should be on their way to medical help. High-dose intravenous corticosteroids and prostacyclin inhibitors have both been used with good results in this setting.

TREATMENT OF RAYNAUD'S

For children with Raynaud's phenomenon without an associated disease, the most important aspect of treatment is common sense. The vast majority of children do well simply by dressing warmly and wearing gloves. If these measures are not enough, children may benefit from the use of calcium-channel blockers (Chapter 20), which block blood vessel constriction. Most children tolerate the mild reduction in blood pressure associated with these drugs without difficulty, but some do get mild side effects. Many of my patients use these drugs only in the coldest weather. In addition to the calcium-channel blockers, it is possible to use drugs such as pentoxifylline. This drug seems to reduce the incidence of Raynaud's, perhaps by making the red blood cell membrane more flexible so it is easier for the cells to get past the area of spasm. Some rheumatologists use aspirin and other agents with varying success.

For children with an underlying rheumatic disease, the key to relieving Raynaud's phenomenon is primarily relief of the underlying condition. In some children with an underlying rheumatic disease, Raynaud's may remain a problem when the majority of the symptoms have resolved. Symptomatic therapy with warm clothing and calcium-channel blockers may be helpful in these cases.

13

Scleroderma

A variety of different diseases are grouped together under the diagnosis of scleroderma. The focal (or localized) forms of scleroderma are often mild and may not require any treatment. In contrast, progressive systemic sclerosis (also called diffuse scleroderma) is a life-threatening disease typically involving the heart, lungs, and other organs. Fortunately, the mild forms of scleroderma are far more common than the severe ones.

LOCALIZED FORMS OF SCLERODERMA

Morphea

Morphea is the most common form of scleroderma in childhood. Morphea consists of areas of thickened skin commonly on the body (trunk), but sometimes on arms or legs. Its cause is unknown. Families usually notice a patch of pink and irritated skin that looks like many common skin conditions. If the patch is due to morphea, it typically does not itch or hurt. Often the area of reddened skin does not attract any particular attention until it has persisted for several weeks. It will not improve with treatment for skin infections, but it might briefly look better if it is treated with corticosteroid creams.

Commonly, the family becomes concerned when either a second area of skin becomes involved or the area begins to enlarge. When areas of morphea are active, they slowly increase in size with the rim remaining pink, but the center turns whitish and becomes hard. Dermatologists usually make the diagnosis of morphea on the basis of either a skin biopsy or clinical experience.

Laboratory abnormalities are rare in children with morphea. Although some children have positive tests for ANA, tests for anti-dsDNA, RF, Scl-70, and anticentromere antibody should be negative, and routine blood tests including complete blood count, erythrocyte sedimentation rate, and muscle enzymes should all be normal. If they are not, a full and complete evaluation by an experienced rheumatologist is in order.

Some lesions of morphea are very small (nickel- or dime-sized), while others can be several inches across. Over a period of years, they usually evolve from hard white areas to soft and darkened skin in light-skinned people; in dark-skinned people the areas of morphea may remain lighter than the surrounding skin. Sometimes this skin is a little sunken relative to the surrounding skin because of loss of the underlying fat. If the morphea is not interfering with function and there are only a few lesions, it may be best to treat it with topical creams such as vitamin E cream or cocoa butter. Chronic use of corticosteroid creams can damage the skin and should be avoided.

Children with rapidly developing morphea lesions that are disfiguring may need aggressive therapy. In my experience, methotrexate therapy has been very successful in stopping the progression of morphea. Low doses of methotrexate given as pills are rarely effective, but moderate doses of methotrexate (1 mg/kg/week, maximum 50 mg) given as subcutaneous injections are very effective. However, the lesions must be significant enough to warrant the risks as well as the time, effort, and expense of therapy. Borderline cases may benefit from treatment with hydroxychloroquine (see Chapter 22).

Morphea has two main complications. First, the lesions are cosmetically unattractive. If they are in a place that is covered by clothing, the problem may be minimal. If the lesions are in a location that is easily seen by others, there will be a need to address the psychological issues associated with the invariable curious questions (see Chapter 24). Second, the skin in the lesions will not heal well if it is cut or abraded.

In rare cases, isolated lesions of morphea may be associated with mild arthritis or other rheumatic disease manifestations. These overlap conditions are of uncertain significance. However, any child with atypical lesions or unexpected problems should be carefully evaluated by an experienced rheumatologist.

Many parents worry that morphea lesions may be the first indications of systemic scleroderma. This is rarely, if ever, true. In most children who develop systemic scleroderma, there is strong evidence suggesting systemic disease from the beginning. If there are no such indications, I recommend only periodic monitoring once the initial evaluation is complete. The long-term outlook for children with morphea is excellent.

Linear Scleroderma

Linear scleroderma differs from morphea in that the areas of involved skin form linear bands instead of irregular ovals. Its cause remains unknown.

A typical case of linear scleroderma in a child presents as a tight band of skin on the top of one foot extending up onto the leg. It may also begin on the hand and arm. These areas appear pinkish at first and don't hurt. Later they become pale and harden. A small area of involvement may be of little concern, but if a large area is involved, tightening of the skin may cause the leg (or arm, toes, etc.) to become bent.

We do not understand the patterns of linear scleroderma. Some children have one patch on one arm or leg. Others have several patches on one arm. Still others may have involvement of both the arm and the leg on one side, and the lesions may extend onto the trunk. Involvement of both sides of the body is unusual and should prompt careful investigation.

Laboratory abnormalities in children with linear scleroderma are minimal. Although some children have positive tests for ANA, tests for anti-dsDNA, RF, Scl-70, anticentromere antibody should be negative, and routine blood tests including CBC and ESR all should be normal. Some children will have mildly elevated muscle enzymes. If a child has elevated muscle enzymes and the typical rash of dermatomyositis in conjunction with an area of linear scleroderma, the disease is termed sclerodermatomyositis (see below).

If the disease occurs while a child is still growing, it may interfere with the development of the underlying muscles, bones, and joints. This may result in an arm or leg that is much smaller than it should be and result in permanent disability. Because of this, areas of linear scleroderma that cross a joint (e.g., elbow, wrist, knee, ankle) require aggressive treatment. Studies have shown excellent success in treating linear scleroderma with methotrexate. Over a six-month period, weekly methotrexate injections are associated with dramatic softening of the skin and reversal of contractures. Although this treatment cannot restore lost muscle or bone mass, it appears to stop the disease and allow further growth in young children. It should be started as soon as possible in children who are developing deformities.

Linear Scleroderma en Coup de Sabre and Parry-Romberg Syndrome

Linear scleroderma en coup de sabre is a particular form of linear scleroderma that may not truly be related to the other forms. Children with linear sclero-derma en coup de sabre have an area of thickened abnormal skin involving one side of the forehead and extending along the scalp toward the back. They usually do not have significant underlying problems.

Parry-Romberg syndrome is a gradually progressive facial hemiatrophy. In a full-fledged case, there is significant deformity, with one entire side of the face smaller than the other. This is in sharp contrast to typical linear scleroderma en coup de sabre, where the abnormality is confined to the forehead. While the changes of linear scleroderma en coup de sabre are usually confined to the skin, in Parry-Romberg syndrome there is an increased frequency of underlying changes in the brain.

The difference between linear scleroderma en coup de sabre and Parry-Romberg syndrome is best exemplified by involvement of the tongue in Parry-Romberg syndrome. Not only is one side of the face smaller, but also one side of the tongue is smaller. Thus, Parry-Romberg syndrome is clearly not a condition of the skin alone. However, both conditions may begin the same way.

These illnesses typically begin in the first or second year of life. Most often the family will describe having noticed a pinkish lesion just to one side of the middle of the forehead. Over a few weeks the lesion does not go away as expected. Instead, the veins may become more noticeable in the pink area.

The lesion on the forehead is often present for months before the family begins to notice indentation of the bone under the pink skin. On careful examination, there may be a continuation of the abnormal skin underneath the hairline. In other children, over time the area of pink skin extends further down the face and along the side of the nose. Linear scleroderma en coup de sabre should not extend below the eyelid. True Parry-Romberg syndrome involves the entire side of the face. Some children fall in between.

Because there are children with varying degrees of involvement, there is no uniform agreement regarding where linear scleroderma en coup de sabre ends and Parry-Romberg syndrome begins. If there is involvement of the tongue, it is Parry-Romberg syndrome. I also believe all children with neurologic involvement have Parry-Romberg syndrome and not linear scleroderma en coup de sabre.

Laboratory abnormalities are minimal in children with both of these disorders. As with other forms of linear scleroderma, some children have positive tests for ANA, but tests for anti-dsDNA, RF, Scl-70, and anticentromere antibody should be negative, and routine blood tests including CBC and ESR should be normal. These children should not have abnormal muscle enzymes or muscle weakness.

Treatment and prognosis for this group of children remain uncertain. If the lesions are confined to the scalp and forehead, as in typical linear scleroderma en coup de sabre, they are responsive to methotrexate. The long-term outlook for children with linear scleroderma en coup de sabre is generally excellent. In most cases the cosmetic deformity is minimal and can be well concealed by the hair.

Unfortunately, children with Parry-Romberg syndrome are rarely recognized before the atrophy has become significant. In most cases, it does not appear appropriate to intervene medically at that point. However, in the hands of an experienced plastic surgeon, cosmetic surgery is practical. There are multiple special considerations involved in this surgery and it should be done only by a team experienced in dealing with such children.

A significant percentage of children with Parry-Romberg syndrome also have underlying central nervous system lesions. These may vary from benign nonspecific findings on MRI to vascular malformations or neurologic abnormalities. I evaluate all children who come to me with Parry-Romberg syndrome with an MRI in order to see whether such abnormalities are present. Some children with Parry-Romberg may have learning disabilities. Although some physicians dismiss this as a coincidence, the association is real.

Some children with Parry-Romberg syndrome have developed inflammation of the optic nerve (the nerve in the back of the eye that provides vision). This is rare but requires immediate treatment if it occurs. I have also cared for children with linear scleroderma en coup de sabre who developed uveitis (ocular inflammation). All children with either linear scleroderma en coup de sabre or Parry-Romberg syndrome should have periodic ophthalmologic evaluations.

The combination of cosmetic and neurologic abnormalities in children with Parry-Romberg syndrome makes the prognosis for these children more guarded. Most do well with corrective surgery. A sympathetic family and physician are important. Special efforts must be made to help these children deal with the social stresses that result from their often obviously abnormal appearance (see Chapter 24).

Sclerodermatomyositis

Sclerodermatomyositis is an overlap disorder in which there is a band of tight skin that appears to be linear scleroderma, but also the muscle weakness, elevated muscle enzymes, and heliotropic rash (a rash in areas exposed to sun, often the face and eyelids) typical of dermatomyositis (see Chapter 14). The simultaneous occurrence of manifestations of two separate diseases in these children is unexplained.

Laboratory abnormalities found in children with sclerodermatomyositis include a positive test for ANA. The routine blood tests may show a mild anemia, elevation of the ESR, and elevated muscle enzyme levels (CK and aldolase; see Chapter 22). RF is rare, and anti-Scl-70 is normally absent. Although diffuse sclerodermatous changes, rash, and elevated muscle enzymes may occur in mixed connective tissue disease, children with MCTD do not have linear bands of tight skin, and the laboratory findings are different.

Complications of sclerodermatomyositis are rare. The muscle inflammation and heliotropic rash most often respond promptly to corticosteroid therapy and do not recur. The linear scleroderma lesion does not respond to corticosteroids, though it may become less pink in coloration. The lesion is rarely large enough to cause concern. If it crosses a joint or causes significant deformity, methotrexate therapy may be necessary. Many children have been treated with long-term hydroxychloroquine once corticosteroids were no longer necessary. Although a small percentage of children will develop further manifestations of rheumatic disease, in general the long-term prognosis is good.

Other Overlapping Conditions

Somehow all of these diseases that look so different in their typical forms are interrelated, but we clearly do not understand the connections. I have seen several children who simultaneously have skin lesions of morphea on their backs and abdomens, indentations typical of linear scleroderma en coup de sabre on their foreheads, ocular inflammation such as that seen in children with juvenile arthritis, and areas of linear scleroderma on their legs. Other overlap conditions may also occur.

The key in caring for children who do not fit neatly into one category or another is to recognize each condition for what it is and treat each appropriately. At the same time, every child presenting with atypical disease must be carefully evaluated to make sure an alternative diagnosis has not been overlooked.

SYSTEMIC FORMS OF SCLERODERMA

Progressive Systemic Sclerosis

The form of scleroderma called progressive systemic sclerosis (PSS), also referred to as diffuse scleroderma, is the most severe form of the disease, with the subtle onset of skin tightening and in many cases shortness of breath. Children and families may be unaware of the disease until it has become well advanced. Because the onset of disease is slow and gradual, families often are unaware of the problem until a dramatic event occurs: a cold and numb finger, the inability to play favorite sports when the season starts, or the inability to open jars or perform other minor chores that the child used to do easily. These children have poor wound healing and may be brought to the physician because of painful sores that do not heal appropriately.

The most common early symptom of PSS is Raynaud's phenomenon. However, it is important to be aware that most people who have Raynaud's phenomenon do not develop rheumatic disease (see Chapter 12). Other common early symptoms of PSS are gradually increasing tightness of the skin and progressive stiffening of the fingers. Typically, these children are ultimately brought to the physician because of shortness of breath, difficulty swallowing, or weight loss.

Diagnosis. An experienced physician easily diagnoses PSS when the skin involvement is prominent. The tight, shiny skin is often accompanied by sores over the knuckles (Gottren's papules), abnormalities in the nail fold capillaries, and distal fingertip lesions (see Chapter 12). This combination of findings is diagnostic of PSS. Less often children come to the doctor because the esophagus is involved and they have difficulty swallowing foods in large chunks or foods that have sharp edges, such as potato chips.

Some children with scleroderma are first seen by their physicians because of chest pain. The distal esophagus is frequently involved in scleroderma, and the valve (sphincter) that keeps stomach acid out of the esophagus often fails to work properly. As a result, the chest pains are due to irritation of the esophagus by acid reflux. Occasionally, children present with chronic diarrhea and weight loss because the intestinal tract is affected by the scleroderma. In all of these cases, the key to the diagnosis is consideration of the possibility of scleroderma by a knowledgeable physician.

Other diseases may be associated with Raynaud's phenomenon or shortness of breath, but the combination of chronic or recurrent shortness of breath and Raynaud's is highly suggestive of PSS or CREST syndrome (see below). MCTD, dermatomyositis, systemic lupus erythematosus, and less frequently other rheumatic diseases may also have both symptoms. Typical cases of MCTD, PSS, and CREST syndrome can be easily differentiated, but there is a broad spectrum of overlap among these diseases. Over time, some children with obvious MCTD progress to having PSS.

The diagnosis of PSS is based on the characteristic findings on examination of the skin. In some cases, it is necessary to biopsy the skin for confirmation, but because the skin of children with scleroderma often heals poorly and the biopsy may produce a scar, it may be best to avoid this where possible.

There are several patterns of laboratory abnormality in children with scleroderma. No single test is abnormal in every child. Frequently, the routine tests (CBC, ESR, chemistry panel) are essentially normal. An increased number of eosinophils may be noted in the blood count. Very high levels of eosinophils may suggest eosinophilic fasciitis (see below). Positive tests for ANA or RF are common but not necessary for the diagnosis. Muscle enzymes (CK, aldolase) may be elevated. Antibodies to Scl-70 (antitopoisomerase antibodies) are less common in children with scleroderma than in adults but may occur. Anti-DNA antibodies are occasionally reported in low titer, but serum complement levels (C3, C4) should be normal.

With the exception of the finding of anti-Scl-70, it may be impossible to differentiate MCTD and PSS on a laboratory basis. Because some children with MCTD ultimately are diagnosed as having evolved into PSS, this may be a false distinction (see Chapter 10). CREST syndrome should be considered carefully in children with telangiectasias or high titers of anticentromere antibody (see section below).

Complications. The most severe complications associated with scleroderma result from involvement of the internal organs. Lung involvement that leads to progressive shortness of breath may be quite severe. Children with PSS should undergo periodic monitoring of their pulmonary function tests (PFTs; see Chapter 22). High-resolution CT scans of the chest are helpful if a child has abnormal PFTs and may be done in children with normal PFTs if there is clinical suspicion of lung disease. Areas of fibrosis indicate significant lung involvement. Over time, this involvement may lead to thickening and loss of elasticity in the lung tissue, much like what happens in the skin. These changes make it harder to move air in and out of the lungs and more difficult for oxygen to move into the blood.

Children with significant lung involvement should be aggressively treated. Over time, the difficulty of moving air in and out of the lungs places additional strain on the heart, which can result in enlargement of the right ventricle, leakage of the pulmonary valve, and increased pulmonary artery pressure. Untreated, severe lung involvement often leads to heart failure, pneumonia, or both.

Some children develop involvement of the heart muscle, known as myocardial fibrosis, which causes the heart to become stiff. It is as if extra fibrous tissue is forming in the heart, just as it does in the skin. When this happens, the heart cannot contract as easily as before. This can be detected by an echocardiogram. It is a very difficult problem to treat. I try to avoid medications such as digitalis that increase the strength of the heart's contractions, because these may cause abnormalities of the heart rhythm. Children with significant cardiac compromise from scleroderma will need an experienced cardiologist to help in their care.

The outer covering of the heart (the pericardium) may also be involved in scleroderma. Most often this takes the form of thickening and irritation (pericarditis), sometimes with a buildup of fluid. If too much fluid is present, it becomes difficult for the heart to pump properly. This can be treated with medications, but if it is very severe, the fluid may need to be drained (pericardiocentesis).

Although children rarely have heart attacks, the coronary arteries may become involved in children with scleroderma. Gradual thickening of the coronary arteries is unlikely to cause problems until the children have become adults. However, some children develop overreactive blood vessels in the heart that constrict when they experience Raynaud's changes in their hands. This should be aggressively treated, as it may result in a heart attack.

Involvement of the kidneys is another major concern for children with PSS. If the blood vessels supplying the kidneys become thickened and narrowed, affecting the pressure in the blood vessels, the kidneys respond by releasing a compound called rennin, which causes the blood pressure to increase throughout the body. In children with scleroderma, the increased blood pressure leads to strain on the heart and other organs. Rarely, children develop an acute rise in blood pressure called scleroderma renal crisis. This is a life-threatening condition. Fortunately, a new class of agents for blood pressure control, the ACE inhibitors, is very effective in treating this problem.

Children with scleroderma frequently have involvement of the gastrointestinal system. Tightness of the skin around the mouth can make it difficult to open the mouth wide enough to eat normally. The thickening of the esophagus may make it difficult to swallow certain foods. In addition, it is common for the valve at the bottom of the esophagus (esophageal sphincter) to lose its ability to close tightly. This results in acid washing up from the stomach (gastroesophageal reflux), causing severe irritation and often resulting in severe chest pain.

Eventually, the gastroesophageal reflux may cause scarring of the esophagus, making it more difficult for food to pass through. Often the pain and discomfort caused by this combination of problems make the child not want to eat, and he or she will begin to lose weight.

When scleroderma involves the intestines, the thickening of the tissues makes it difficult for the intestines to move food forward in the normal fashion. The result is poor absorption of nutrients and chronic bloating. Some patients have problems with constipation, others have problems with diarrhea, and some have both. These digestive problems frequently worsen the child's weight loss.

Liver involvement in children with scleroderma is rare. Some cases of primary biliary cirrhosis (an uncommon form of liver disease) have been reported.

Treatment. Proper treatment of childhood scleroderma remains controversial. However, it is generally agreed that treatment with D-penicillamine (which used to be the standard therapy) is ineffective. There is no clear agreement on the best treatment for mild cases. Some feel short courses of prednisone are helpful. I personally avoid them if possible.

The key to obtaining the best outcome for children with scleroderma is to prevent severe internal organ involvement. Most physicians will treat children with systemic scleroderma with mild agents such as hydroxychloroquine unless there is severe internal organ involvement. If that is present, they will treat the children with intravenous cyclophosphamide. My own preference is to treat every child with definite PSS with injections of methotrexate (1 mg/kg per week) and oral cyclosporine.

A variety of medications have been tried in adults with scleroderma. The use of TNF inhibitors and agents that block B cell activity (such as rituximab) is being considered. See Chapter 20 for a fuller discussion of these medications.

An assortment of medications is used to address specific problems. As noted, ACE inhibitors are used to treat increased blood pressure. Calcium-channel blockers are used to treat Raynaud's phenomenon. Any of several medicines that block acid secretion can be used to minimize damage to the esophagus. In addition, prostaglandins such as inhaled iloprost have been used to treat pulmonary fibrosis and the resultant increase in stiffness of the blood vessels in the lungs. There is no single best therapy, but it is important for parents to make sure that their children are being followed by physicians who are familiar with the most current recommendations. Children with significant PSS should be cared for at major medical centers with experienced rheumatologists, pulmonologists, cardiologists, nephrologists, and specialists in intensive care—preferably with extensive pediatric experience. The primary goal must be to prevent progression of the disease.

Prognosis. The prognosis for children with PSS is guarded. In the absence of significant internal organ involvement, children may live for decades. Some children with only skin involvement may find that their skin eventually softens and will do well. Children with significant heart, lung, kidney, or gastrointestinal involvement did poorly in the past. However, with more aggressive therapy the outlook is improving. There is reason to believe that continued aggressive treatment will allow children with PSS to lead reasonably normal lives.

CREST Syndrome

CREST syndrome is a variation of systemic scleroderma that has several peculiar aspects. The name *CREST* is an acronym that comes from the findings of calcinosis (pieces of calcium under the skin), Raynaud's phenomenon, esophageal problems, sclerodactyly (tight skin on the fingers), and telangiectasias (small red spots due to abnormal blood vessels in the skin). The key findings that distinguish CREST from PSS are the presence of telangiectasias and anticentromere antibodies.

The general problems associated with CREST syndrome and their treatments do not differ from PSS. However, it is clear that these children are somehow different from the children with PSS. Often these children have less skin and kidney involvement but more heart and lung involvement. Treatment is essentially the same for CREST and PSS.

EOSINOPHILIC FASCIITIS: A DISEASE THAT CAN EVOLVE INTO SCLERODERMA

Eosinophilic fasciitis is an unusual disorder characterized by the acute onset of pain and swelling in an extremity. It is named for the fact that in affected individuals, the connective tissue, or fascia, is inflamed (fasciitis) and there is an abundance of eosinophils (a white blood cell type associated with allergies and not commonly present in the fascia). Typically, the skin in the affected area is very red, tender, and swollen. This inflammation is followed by hardening of the skin and muscles in the area. Although the onset of eosinophilic fasciitis is commonly associated with extreme exercise or trauma, the cause is poorly understood. Evidence of inflammation, including an increased sedimentation rate and increased eosinophil count, are common. Internal organ involvement does not occur.

Some cases of eosinophilic myalgia syndrome were initially thought to be eosinophilic fasciitis. This is a syndrome with muscle pain and redness but not fasciitis. In the late 1980s, an epidemic of eosinophilic myalgia was apparently caused by contaminated L-tryptophan supplements.

Eosinophilic fasciitis is usually very responsive to treatment with corticosteroids. However, the long-term course of the disease is highly varied. Sometimes the disease resolves entirely, but other cases persist with varying amounts of disease activity for years. A few children have ultimately developed PSS after initially being diagnosed with eosinophilic fasciitis. However, most cases have resolved completely over a period of months.

Children with eosinophilia and musculoskeletal complaints need to be evaluated very carefully. This combination of findings may occur in children with parasitic illnesses, eosinophilic vasculitis, and Churg-Strauss disease. These diseases are uncommon but may be life-threatening if not properly recognized and treated. Children with these diseases may have rashes, but these diseases are not associated with hardening of the skin.

14

Dermatomyositis and Polymyositis

Dermatomyositis in childhood is characterized by weakness of the proximal muscles (those muscles closest to the trunk) and rash. In most cases the disease begins slowly, with the gradual onset of progressive weakness. However, a small percentage of cases begin with dramatic fever, rash, elevated muscle enzymes, and profound weakness. Dermatomyositis may begin in any age group, sometimes affecting very young children and at other times teenagers. The dermatomyositis that occurs in adults appears to be different from the disease in childhood. The key to the diagnosis of dermatomyositis is recognition of progressive muscle weakness involving the upper arms and upper legs to a much greater degree than the hands and feet. It is always associated with a rash, usually on the upper eyelids and over the elbows and knees.

Polymyositis is extremely rare in childhood. The key factor differentiating it from dermatomyositis is the absence of rash. Children with polymyositis have the same pattern of proximal muscle weakness as is seen in children with dermatomyositis. This is a rare condition and its natural history is unclear. In what follows, I will refer to dermatomyositis for a child who has polymyositis.

There are a number of illnesses that may cause muscle weakness in children. In addition to dermatomyositis, the gradual onset of weakness in small children can come from botulinum spores (found in honey and possibly other unpasteurized or improperly processed foods), intrinsic muscle diseases including muscular dystrophy, and a variety of metabolic diseases. The abrupt onset of muscle weakness may occur with viral infections, poisoning by insecticides and other toxic substances, certain venomous snakebites, and some medications. During some flu epidemics many children will complain of pain in their calves and have elevated muscle enzyme levels. The key finding that differentiates dermatomyositis from these conditions is the presence of rash and different patterns of muscle weakness. Children with dermatomyositis are weak everywhere, but the thighs and upper arms are much weaker than expected when compared with the hands and feet.

In children with dermatomyositis, hand and foot strength are relatively good (though they may be less than normal), while the ability to raise the hands over the head (e.g., when brushing the hair) and to raise the legs (e.g., when going upstairs) is clearly reduced. Any child of an appropriate age who cannot raise the arms over the head, get up easily from a chair, or get up off the floor without assistance should be evaluated by an experienced physician.

The diagnosis of dermatomyositis is made on the basis of the history and the physical examination findings plus appropriate blood tests. Either the creatine kinase (CK) or the aldolase level will be abnormal in most children with dermatomyositis. These tests indicate muscle inflammation, but they can also be abnormal following viral infections or extensive physical activity (e.g., playing football, running track, lifting weights). Often these tests are not included in the routine chemistry panel and have to be specifically ordered by the physician. All of the routine tests, including the erythrocyte sedimentation rate, might be normal despite active dermatomyositis.

Absolute proof of dermatomyositis requires a muscle biopsy demonstrating the death of muscle cells with a characteristic pathologic pattern (perifascicular infiltration of inflammatory cells). The diagnosis can also be made if electromyography (EMG) demonstrates a characteristic "spike and wave" pattern. The muscle biopsy and EMG must be done on the inflamed muscle. Biopsy of an uninvolved muscle may lead to a false negative pathology report.

Before a muscle biopsy is done it is often useful to obtain an MRI of the thighs. Inflamed muscles are swollen and show up on the MRI because they have greater water content than uninvolved muscles. Once the MRI has demonstrated the presence of inflamed muscles in a weak child, a muscle biopsy may not need to be done unless another cause of muscle inflammation is suspected; the diagnosis may be made on the basis of a characteristic history and examination findings with confirmatory laboratory tests. Children with dermatomyositis frequently have poor skin healing, and a biopsy may leave a significant scar.

Children who have a rash typical of dermatomyositis and mildly elevated muscle enzymes but no evident weakness require particular attention. These children clearly have the disease; the elevated muscle enzymes and rash are evidence of ongoing inflammation and damage. Rather than wait for things to get worse, I believe it is important to treat these children appropriately to bring the muscle inflammation under control. Often these children require only a short course of therapy and do well.

There are several subtypes of dermatomyositis that have been recognized. The most common form of dermatomyositis is typically referred to as unicyclic or monocyclic. This form of dermatomyositis most often occurs in small children. There is gradual onset of weakness and rash. These children do not have nail fold capillary abnormalities, poorly healing skin, or inflammation over the knuckles.

Children with polycyclic disease usually have the same initial symptoms as the children with unicyclic disease, but these children often do have nail fold capillary abnormalities, inflammation over their knuckles, and in some cases poorly healing skin. It is important to recognize that these children are different from the first group of children. They will require more aggressive therapy for a longer period and remain vulnerable to relapses.

Children with polycyclic disease may have several recurrences of muscle inflammation over a period of two or three years. At the end of that period, they may be left with complications secondary to the development of calcifications or other internal organ involvement (see "Complications of Dermatomyositis," below), but active muscle inflammation is less common.

Some children with dermatomyositis have chronic recurrent disease. The relationship of this form of the disease to the other forms is unclear. Children with chronic recurrent dermatomyositis often appear more ill during the acute phase of their illness. Their muscle enzyme levels are often very high and do not seem to respond significantly to therapy. Vasculitis is a common component of this form of the disease.

There is increasing recognition of a group of patients with a disease that resembles dermatomyositis. They have muscle involvement, abnormal antibodies to tRNA synthetase (Jo-1) and related molecules, and an increased frequency of lung involvement and other problems. Most of the patients like this have been adults; the antibodies to Jo-1 are very infrequent in children. If they are present, more careful evaluation is required and more aggressive treatment may be necessary. It is not clear this is the same disease as dermatomyositis.

COMPLICATIONS OF DERMATOMYOSITIS

Complications of properly treated unicyclic dermatomyositis are usually minor. There are two important types of complications that occur more frequently in children with polycyclic disease. Vasculitis (inflammation of the blood vessels) in the skin and muscles is characteristic of this form of the disease. Its presence is strongly suggested by the occurrence of nail fold capillary abnormalities and inflammation over the knuckles. In some children, there also may be vasculitis of the intestines, which can produce severe abdominal pain and serious intestinal complications. Any child with dermatomyositis who has chronic or recurrent abdominal pain must be investigated very carefully. Vasculitis-related complications can also occur in other organ systems, including the central nervous system, lungs, and kidneys. Children with these complications are at significant risk and require aggressive therapy to minimize the chance of a poor outcome.

The second important type of complication that occurs more frequently in children with polycyclic disease is the development of subcutaneous or intramuscular calcifications. These calcifications, which are easily seen in X-rays, appear as the muscle inflammation is disappearing and may be thought of as a scarring response. Unfortunately, they may cause major problems. Infection often occurs when the calcifications have formed over the elbows or other points where they are constantly being irritated by pressure. They may spontaneously become swollen and tender, and then drain to the outside. The initial drainage most often is not infected, but once leakage to the outside occurs, there is a significant risk that the draining lesion will become infected. Large calcifications within the musculature may become infected as well. They may also be a source of ongoing muscular irritation. In some cases these calcifications may disappear over time, but there is little that can be done for existing ones. Surgeons sometimes remove large calcifications, but this may be associated with poor wound healing and significant long-term problems. There have been some recent reports describing substantial improvement of severe calcifications after treatment with bisphosphonates (drugs that prevent the withdrawal of calcium from the bones), but the best therapy for calcifications is to prevent their occurrence by providing prompt diagnosis and treatment for children with dermatomyositis.

Permanent loss of strength may occur when large numbers of muscle cells die during the inflammatory phase of dermatomyositis. While with use individual muscle cells may grow larger, increasing strength, we do not make new muscle cells to replace ones that are lost. Our bodies have significant reserves of muscle cells, but if too many are lost, a child will never be able to recover full strength. Again, prompt diagnosis and treatment are essential to the best outcome.

In addition to these more common complications, there are rare complications related to vasculitis of the central nervous system (brain) in some cases of severe polycyclic disease. This can result in psychological disturbances, hallucinations, and even seizures. Children with these complications must be treated aggressively. The kidneys are also involved in some children with polycyclic or chronic recurrent disease. This may result in blood or protein in the urine (hematuria or proteinuria). Normally, this is not serious and does not lead to significant damage to the kidneys.

Lipodystrophy is a more unusual complication seen in some children with dermatomyositis. This condition is associated with widespread loss of subcutaneous fat. Some children have lesser areas of involvement (localized or partial lipodystrophy). Children with generalized lipodystrophy appear very thin. Characteristic of the loss of subcutaneous fat is the ability to easily see the blood vessels through the skin. Even in its partial form, this condition may be associated with abnormal lipid metabolism and diabetes with insulin resistance. Lipodystrophy is seen in other rheumatic diseases, and its relationship to the diagnosis of dermatomyositis is unclear. Children with this condition will need to be under the care of a multidisciplinary team in an experienced center.

TREATMENT OF DERMATOMYOSITIS

The type of disease, the degree of weakness, and the nature of the complications determine the medical treatment of dermatomyositis.

As noted previously, I believe that children who have a rash typical of dermatomyositis and mildly elevated muscle enzymes but no weakness should be treated. They clearly do have inflammation, and there is no sense in waiting for enough muscle cells to die to make it obvious they are weak before we begin to treat them.

For children without evidence of vasculitis who are not profoundly weak, a low or moderate dose of corticosteroids is often sufficient. Some children with dermatomyositis have mild arthritis when they first come to a doctor's attention. This usually responds well to treatment with corticosteroids, but a brief course of nonsteroidal anti-inflammatory drugs (NSAIDs) may also be beneficial. Hydroxychloroquine is another drug that is often useful as a steroid-sparing agent in children with mild disease, especially where rash predominates.

Children with evidence of vasculitis (nail fold capillary abnormalities, poor wound healing, changes of the skin over the knuckles) often respond well to a moderate dose of corticosteroids. Typically, as the corticosteroids are withdrawn, these children develop recurrent problems. When this is the case, the addition of methotrexate is often beneficial. Alternative regimens include the use of cyclosporine, intravenous gamma globulin, or—for severe methotrexate-resistant disease— cyclophosphamide. Rituximab has been successful in treating dermatomyositis when added to therapy with cyclophosphamide or methotrexate.

Severe weakness needs to be treated. In particular, if a child has developed a nasal voice or has begun to cough when eating, immediate intervention with high-dose corticosteroids is vital. These findings suggest weakness of the muscles needed for swallowing and thus indicate a risk of aspiration (food going into the lungs), which can be disastrous.

Children with chronic recurrent dermatomyositis frequently require treatment with corticosteroids and methotrexate but may respond only incompletely. Fortunately, they are rarely as weak as their laboratory values would suggest.

Over the long term, persistent weakness and secondary calcifications remain the most distressing problems for children with dermatomyositis. Rapid diagnosis and appropriate treatment minimize the amount of muscle cell death. Since calcification in the skin and musculature is a healing response, early aggressive therapy is also the best means of preventing this problem.

Physical therapy to maintain range of motion and maximize the strength of the remaining musculature is a major component of care for children with dermatomyositis. During the period when there is active muscle inflammation, the therapist should concentrate on passive range of motion. Only after the muscle inflammation has been controlled should active exercises begin.

In general, surgical therapy is not a significant component of the care of children with dermatomyositis. Excision and drainage of infected calcifications may be necessary in some children. Poor wound healing limits the utility of surgical efforts to remove large calcifications. Children with inflammation of the vessels that supply blood to the intestines may require urgent surgical intervention.

PROGNOSIS FOR CHILDREN WITH DERMATOMYOSITIS

The prognosis for most children with dermatomyositis is very good. Most children have unicyclic disease and do well. With early diagnosis and prompt therapy, most children with polycyclic disease also have a good outcome. An experienced medical team can usually handle recurrent infections of subcutaneous calcifications without major problems, provided the patient seeks care promptly. Most parents should regard dermatomyositis as a very treatable condition with an excellent prognosis.

Children with polycyclic disease associated with significant complications because of inflammation of the blood vessels supplying internal organs have a more guarded prognosis. This is also true for children who have lost substantial numbers of muscle cells or suffered significant intramuscular calcifications. These children should be referred to specialized centers where the best possible efforts can be made to avoid what is sometimes a very poor outcome. These cases are often the result of delayed diagnosis or inadequate therapy. The long-term prognosis for children with chronic recurrent dermatomyositis is uncertain.

Recurrent lung infections resulting from excessive muscle loss leading to difficulty in coughing and maintaining respiration occur only in the most severe cases. It may not be possible to restore function to all of these children, and infection is a serious risk. Fortunately, such cases have become rare. With prompt diagnosis and treatment, the majority of children with dermatomyositis will do well.

15

Kawasaki Disease

Kawasaki disease usually begins in a young child as fever and irritability without apparent explanation. Within the first few days, some children develop a swollen lymph node below the jaw. Usually this is thought to be a bacterial infection and is treated with antibiotics. Young children with high fevers who do not develop a swollen lymph node are frequently begun on antibiotics for presumed ear infections. Some children already have a rash at this point, but often the child will develop a rash the next day that may be confused with an allergy to the antibiotic.

Physicians usually do not begin to think about Kawasaki disease (KD) until the child continues with fever and rash even after the antibiotics. In a typical case, the child will develop inflammation of the eyes (which may look red or bloodshot) and dry cracked red lips or an irritated tongue over the next few days of illness. Also about this time the hands and feet often become diffusely swollen. Laboratory tests indicate the white blood cell count is going up, and so are the erythrocyte sedimentation rate and the platelet count, sometimes to very high levels. At this point the physician may recognize KD. However, early diagnosis of KD is difficult because many serious infections, including measles and severe streptococcal infections, can look just like KD at the very beginning.

The cause of Kawasaki disease is not well understood. The disease tends to occur in epidemics, which suggests that it is an infection. However, infections usually spread among children in the same household, and for KD it is rare to find a second child in the same household or a playmate with the disease. However, there is evidence that KD is spread by exposure to some type of agent. KD is more common in areas that have been recently flooded and in households where the carpets have recently been shampooed, suggesting that dampness may play a role. Investigations of viruses, fungi, and bacteria have not turned up any clear cause. It is likely that KD is not a common result of an uncommon agent, but the uncommon result of a common agent. This would explain the disease's predilection for young children and occurrence in epidemics.

DIAGNOSIS OF KAWASAKI DISEASE

The most important aspect of the diagnosis and treatment of KD is prompt recognition of the disease. However, there are a variety of illnesses that may produce a similar appearance. It is very important to be sure that the child is not suffering from a significant infection. Measles, streptococcal infections, drug reactions, and many forms of vasculitis may result in a clinical picture that satisfies the criteria for a diagnosis of KD. Hemolytic uremic syndrome has also been confused with KD.

There is a significant concern that children diagnosed with atypical KD in fact have another illness. Coronary artery aneurysms (see "Complications of Kawasaki Disease," below) may occur in children with a number of rheumatic diseases, including polyarteritis nodosa (inflammation of the arteries) and Takayasu's arteritis (inflammation of the aorta). Further, thickening of the coronary arteries on echocardiogram is a nonspecific finding, occurring in many other conditions, and should not be used to establish a diagnosis of KD.

Laboratory findings in KD typically include a dramatically rising white blood cell count, erythrocyte sedimentation rate, and platelet count. Failure of any of these indices to rise appropriately by the seventh day of illness should raise suspicion that the child does not in fact have KD. A falling platelet count is never consistent with the diagnosis of KD unless there are severe complicating factors. Although small amounts of red and white blood cells may appear in the urine, significant kidney involvement is not a normal manifestation of KD.

COMPLICATIONS OF KAWASAKI DISEASE

Once the diagnosis of KD has been properly established, the major concern is whether the child has any cardiac involvement. Early in the illness, a small number of children develop inflammation of the muscles of the heart (pancarditis). Some children develop a coronary artery aneurysm (a bulge in the wall of an artery near the heart). The risk is that the bulge may fill with clotted blood, blocking blood flow and causing a heart attack. Fortunately, this is rare. The second major concern is that the area of the coronary artery damaged by the aneurysm may heal in a way that predisposes the child to heart problems years later. Children with very large coronary artery aneurysms (greater than 8 mm) early in KD have a high frequency of cardiac problems and should be cared for at an advanced center, and all children with aneurysms should be followed up by a cardiologist. A small number of children with KD develop aneurysms in other arteries of the body. These aneurysms may cause problems either during the initial illness or later. Fortunately, most children with KD have no aneurysms or only thickening of the coronary arteries on echocardiogram. This thickening is often not meaningful and can be seen in children who are sick with other conditions.

Some children with KD have less common symptoms. One well-described pattern is the child with severe abdominal pain who has gallbladder involvement found on abdominal ultrasound. Severe headaches and neck pain are also well described but less common. Some children with KD develop aseptic meningitis; if there is significant pain, a spinal tap may be necessary to make sure the child does not have bacterial meningitis, which must be treated immediately. Arthritis with pain and swelling of the knees occurs in some children with KD. Other uncommon findings include inflammation of the pancreas, the kidneys, and the urinary tract.

TREATMENT OF KAWASAKI DISEASE

Once the diagnosis of KD is established, the antibiotics can be stopped and appropriate anti-inflammatory therapy started. Intravenous IgG is usually given right away because it very quickly stops the inflammation associated with KD. The early administration of IV IgG (within ten days of the onset of symptoms) has been shown to dramatically reduce the risk of developing coronary artery aneurysms. If physicians are unsure of the diagnosis but want to treat with IgG, they should save a tube of blood for any later tests that are needed, as IgG contains pooled antibodies from many different people and once it has been given, serologic testing to look for other explanations for the child's illness will be unreliable for many weeks.

Some physicians mistakenly believe IV IgG should be given only during the first ten days of illness. This is wrong. While the efficacy of IgG in preventing aneurysms when given after the tenth day has not been studied, it is safe and does an excellent job of controlling the inflammation associated with KD.

The less common complications of KD, including gallbladder involvement, headaches, neck pain, aseptic meningitis, arthritis of the knees, and inflammation of the pancreas, kidneys, or urinary tract usually respond to therapy for the KD and in most cases do not require special treatment.

In children with typical Kawasaki disease, IgG treatment is followed quickly by an end to the fever and prompt improvement in other symptoms. Occasionally, children require a second dose of IV IgG. Any child who is not better after two doses of IV IgG should be carefully reevaluated. I have seen children with poly-arteritis nodosa, systemic-onset JA, and other rheumatic diseases and infections mistakenly diagnosed as having KD. They do not get better with IV IgG or improve only briefly.

In the absence of infection or other contraindication, corticosteroids may be given to children who have not responded to IV IgG. Although there are reported cases of children with KD improving significantly, then relapsing a few days later, this is rare. There are also reports of children having had KD twice, with months to years separating the episodes. These recurrences are very infrequent.

16

Benign Hypermobile Joint Syndrome and Ehlers-Danlos Syndrome

The role of the ligaments is to maintain the joints in proper position with respect to each other. If they are loose, they don't perform this function properly. Children with either benign hypermobile joint syndrome or Ehlers-Danlos syndrome have loose ligaments, but that is where the similarity ends. Benign hypermobile joint syndrome is not really a disease at all. Instead, it is an inherited variation on normal, and children with benign hypermobile joint syndrome are often referred to as double-jointed. By contrast, children with Ehlers-Danlos syndrome have a defect in their collagen that causes the loosening of the ligaments. Confusion may arise because some physicians refer to benign hypermobile joint syndrome with the term *Ehlers-Danlos type III*, but they are not the same thing.

BENIGN HYPERMOBILE JOINT SYNDROME

The diagnosis of benign hypermobile joint syndrome requires that a child be able to do each of the following:

- Bend the fingers back over the wrist so that they are parallel with the forearm (i.e., they point straight backward)
- Easily bend the thumb back to touch the forearm
- Fully extend the elbow all the way beyond straight (hyperextension)
- Fully extend the knee beyond straight
- Bend over and touch the palms to the floor with the knees straight

The ability to bend joints to a greater than normal degree does not normally seem to be a handicap. Indeed, many children with benign hypermobile joint syndrome, especially girls, are extremely good gymnasts. They can easily do splits and other gymnastic activities that others have difficulty with.

This flexibility comes at a cost, however. In children with benign hypermobile joint syndrome, the loose ligaments allow the bones on each side of the joint to knock into each other repeatedly. Over time this leads to damage to the bones and joints that may become quite severe. The key is to recognize the syndrome and allow the children to reduce their activity and minimize the damage.

Most often the children I see with benign hypermobile joint syndrome are ten- or eleven-year-old girls who take gymnastics or ballet but are beginning to complain of pain in their knees or other joints after practice. This can result from overuse of normal joints, but the child with lax ligaments is likely to have problems that occur earlier and are more severe. For many children the symptoms begin at seven or eight years of age but are dismissed as a minor overuse injury. If the activity has been continued despite the pain, there may be joint swelling and pain on compression of the bones around the joint. Sustained activity can lead to permanent damage

Complications of Benign Hypermobile Joint Syndrome

Significant complications of benign hypermobile joint syndrome are very rare. However, the same material that makes up ligaments also makes up internal structures such as the aortic root, the ring of tissue that connects the aorta (the large main blood vessel that carries blood to the rest of the body) to the heart. If a child has very lax ligaments, he or she should have an echocardiogram done to look for any loosening of the aortic root. If this ring tears, it can cause a rip to form in the aorta, leading to sudden death. It is important to note that this does not happen to children with benign hypermobile joint syndrome, but some children with Ehlers-Danlos syndrome are mistakenly thought to have only benign hypermobile joint syndrome.

Treatment of Benign Hypermobile Joint Syndrome

The joint pains and irritation associated with benign hypermobile joint syndrome can be relieved with mild nonsteroidal anti-inflammatory drugs (NSAIDs), but the key to proper treatment is minimizing the activity until the body matures further.

Physical therapy is often useful to strengthen the muscles around the joint. Surgery is necessary only if severe joint damage has occurred, which is rarely the case. Surgery intended to prevent the bone from repeatedly popping out of the joint is usually not successful because children with benign hypermobile joint syndrome have collagen that is genetically weaker than normal, and surgery cannot correct that.

EHLERS-DANLOS SYNDROME

The classical presentation of Ehlers-Danlos syndrome is in a child who is tall (usually thin) with long arms, long legs, and long thin fingers (children with Marfan's syndrome may also have some of these characteristics). These children have a severe defect in their collagen and are easily recognized because it is easy to stretch their skin. If these children have a cut, it will heal poorly and the scars often become unusually large and thin. By the time they are ten or eleven years old, these children have often had multiple orthopedic problems because of the loose ligaments.

The evaluation of children in whom Ehlers-Danlos syndrome is suspected should include an echocardiogram to evaluate the aortic root (see "Complications of Benign Hypermobile Joint Syndrome," above).

17

Fibromyalgia and Chronic Fatigue Syndrome

Fibromyalgia and chronic fatigue syndrome are complex diseases, and a complete and thorough diagnostic evaluation is essential for any child suspected of having either of these conditions.

FIBROMYALGIA

Children with fibromyalgia complain of widespread pain and fatigue that interfere with normal activities and often cause them to miss many days of school. These children have often been to a variety of physicians without a definitive diagnosis. The generally accepted criteria for a diagnosis of fibromyalgia require widespread pain (above and below the waist and on both the right and left sides) and the presence of at least eleven of eighteen defined "trigger points" (areas that when stimulated give rise to pain in other parts of the body).

Onset often follows a severe viral infection or an injury, and in the majority of cases it seems as though the child never fully recovered from the infection or injury. A number of explanations have been proposed for the continuing pain and fatigue suffered by these children, mostly emphasizing the increased sensitivity of the nervous system, whether because of damaged nerve conduction pathways, altered hormonal balance, persisting infectious agents, or another cause, but none has provided the scientific basis for consistently useful therapy.

The first thing to do in such circumstances is to take a complete history and do a thorough physical and laboratory evaluation to find out whether something has been missed. Often this will yield an unsuspected clue. However, in many cases, no explanation is found.

CHRONIC FATIGUE SYNDROME

Chronic fatigue syndrome (CFS) differs from fibromyalgia because the patients lack the typical trigger points associated with fibromyalgia. Like fibromyalgia, chronic fatigue syndrome is not associated with laboratory abnormalities, a known cause, or a known cure.

Once the diagnosis of CFS has been established and other significant medical problems have been excluded, children with chronic fatigue syndrome should be rehabilitated just as I describe for fibromyalgia in the next section.

TREATMENT OF FIBROMYALGIA AND CHRONIC FATIGUE SYNDROME

My approach to treating children with fibromyalgia and CFS emphasizes rehabilitation and return to activities of daily living. If one views recovery from either of these conditions as one would view recovery from a major physical injury, the steps make good sense. The child, family, and physicians must recognize that there will not be a sudden, miraculous recovery. Progress is made through a rigorous program of slow and steadily increasing level of activities. It is important for every member of the team to acknowledge the reality of the initial problem and the psychological difficulty of dealing with it.

Some children recover well with time, reassurance, medications, and support from their family and doctors. For more difficult cases, a hospital-based team approach is often beneficial. The team in a large children's rehabilitation center consists of nurses, physical and occupational therapists, social workers, psychologists, and pediatricians. Once the diagnosis of fibromyalgia or CFS has been confirmed, it is important for the family to meet with all the appropriate members of the team. Even while this is being done, the family can take the first steps toward recovery.

Getting Back on Schedule

Anyone who has traveled overseas and suffered jet lag can immediately relate to the impact of disordered sleep patterns that is typical of fibromyalgia and CFS. Just as the key to overcoming jet lag is to promptly begin to set your body's wake/sleep cycle on the appropriate schedule for the time zone you are in, families must start children back on a regular schedule of getting up at an appropriate time in the morning (the same time as if they were going off to school normally). This should be accompanied by a policy that lights, computers, televisions, video games, and so on must be turned off at the appropriate time for a school night. Do not expect instant success; it can take two to three weeks or more to adjust to the new schedule. However, if the child gets up at the appropriate time in the morning, it becomes easier and easier to fall asleep at the appropriate time and sleep through the night.

Increasing Physical Activity

Even as the child is adjusting to getting up at the appropriate time each morning, it is important to begin a program of gradually increasing physical activity. For children in the rehabilitation center, this is done under the supervision of a physical therapist. For children being treated as outpatients, this may not be necessary if they are attending school. Children who are not attending school will need regularly scheduled physical therapy at least three days a week with parent-supervised physical activity on the other days.

Too often families overreach in this initial physical therapy. While there are special supervised programs that "jump-start" children with severe disease under carefully supervised circumstances, intense therapy is not appropriate for everyone. A child who has been incapacitated for a prolonged period will need to start exercising slowly. At first, three or four sessions of exercise lasting only fifteen minutes each may be all the child is capable of in a given day. Significant muscular discomfort normally accompanies the resumption of activities in someone who has been disabled for a prolonged period. This discomfort may be treated with NSAIDs, topical creams for sore muscles, and massage. The key to the success of this program is that it be continued despite the muscle soreness and related complaints.

Physical and Occupational Therapy

Physical and occupational therapy play a vital role in the care of children with severe fibromyalgia. Just as a child severely injured in an auto accident would never be expected to recover without physical therapy, a child with severe fibromyalgia or CFS should not be expected to do it on his or her own, either. The key is finding a therapist who understands that the injury in fibromyalgia is every bit as real as the injury to the child who was in an accident.

The program of slowly increasing physical activities to improve strength and endurance must be tailored to the disability level of the child. Over a period of three months it should be possible to gradually increase the level of physical activity to the point where the child feels capable of returning to school, though for some children it may take longer. In all cases, however, the goal should be a full recovery.

Psychological and Emotional Support

During the initial weeks of establishing a program of consistent wake/sleep hours and exercise, it is normal for the child to increase his or her complaints at certain points and the parents to become discouraged. Psychological and emotional support from the family and the psychologist treating the child is critical at this point. Antidepressant medications may be necessary for some children during this stage.

At the beginning of the program, children will experience difficulty adjusting their sleep schedule and resuming physical activity. There is frequently another period of difficulty and resistance six to eight weeks into the program. Children often decide, "This is not working and I'm tired of it." Just as we would never allow a child to give up on recovering after being in a car accident, we cannot let these children give up on recovering, either. These periods of stress and frustration are a normal part of every recovery, and both parents and children should expect them. The physical and emotional pain of trying to do a little more every day is often best dealt with by solid physical, emotional, and psychological support.

The loss of strength and endurance that occurs in fibromyalgia is accompanied by the loss of self-confidence and self-esteem. If a child had major injuries from a car accident and had bad dreams or was afraid to enter another car, no one would be embarrassed to ask for psychological help. Unfortunately, because we do not understand what happened to them, children with fibromyalgia often do not get the sympathetic support given to children with obvious injuries. From a psychological point of view, this makes the situation much worse for children with fibromyalgia. A sympathetic family, physician, and psychologist or psychiatrist are all very important.

Expect a Relapse

Some children will relapse within four to six weeks of returning to school and a full, normal schedule. The rehabilitation team routinely anticipates this setback. Children are so anxious to succeed that they often push themselves beyond their limits during their first days back. Depending on the situation, the rehabilitation team may choose initially to have the child restart school on a part-time basis in order to avoid this problem. This is a decision that should be made by the entire team working together.

Periodic relapse or fear of relapse in association with viral infections and other stresses may occur. The key to successful management of these episodes is for the child and family to pull together and keep things on track. While it may be necessary to spend twenty-four to forty-eight hours in bed with the flu, it is essential that children with a history of fibromyalgia promptly get themselves back on their feet and resume normal activity. The attitude of the rehabilitation team and family must be one of steady reassurance and support for the child.

Equally important in the care of children with fibromyalgia is recognition of the needs of the other family members (see Chapter 24). The stress on other family members of dealing with a child's serious illness can feed back and affect the child him- or herself. This is why it is important that the entire family, including parents and siblings, be involved in the educational activities and psychological counseling that are part of the rehabilitation process. Too often other family members view the sensitivity of the child with fibromyalgia or CFS as manipulative behavior. All must realize that these are not self-induced illnesses and the child really does want to get better. Such complex dynamics can be properly dealt with only if the entire family is willing to participate in the process.

Medical Treatment

While medications are a key component of therapy for adults with fibromyalgia or CFS, they are less important in children. However, NSAIDs, including tramadol, may be helpful in controlling the aches and pains associated with activity. Pregabalin is a medication that has been approved for the treatment of fibromyalgia. It reduces the transmission of nervous impulses carrying the sensation of pain. It certainly helps, but it is not "magic." Amitriptyline is an antidepressant that has been found to have beneficial effects for children and adults with fibromyalgia beyond the antidepressant effect. Children who are greatly troubled by muscle spasm often benefit from the addition of cyclobenzaprine or a similar agent.

Opiate pain medications must be used carefully, if at all. They do not relieve any symptoms other than pain. They frequently cause nausea, worsen sleep patterns, increase ones' overall sense of ill health, and interfere with school attendance and normal life.

PROGNOSIS FOR CHILDREN WITH FIBROMYALGIA OR CHRONIC FATIGUE SYNDROME

The prognosis for children with fibromyalgia or chronic fatigue syndrome who get proper care is excellent. However, just as a child left to languish in bed after suffering serious injury in a car accident would do poorly, so will a child who is left to languish with fibromyalgia or CFS. There is no reason that a child with fibromyalgia or CFS should not be able to be rehabilitated and to resume a fully productive life.

18

Reflex Sympathetic Dystrophy

Reflex sympathetic dystrophy (RSD), reflex neurovascular dystrophy, and complex regional pain syndrome are all various names for the same condition. It is a cause of great frustration for parents and physicians, and it is far more common than you might think. RSD can involve the foot or hand. It rarely occurs in children under the age of eight, but may occur at any age thereafter.

Because there is virtually always a well-documented history of injury preceding the chronic pain, families and physicians are often distraught over their inability to fix the problem. The key to understanding RSD is to recognize that the problem is no longer a simple physical injury. Children with RSD are very often overachievers who have been put under too much pressure to perform—for example, a talented figure skater who makes it all the way to the regional championships but takes a fall and, despite proper orthopedic treatment, is unable to put any weight on the foot, or sometimes even is unable to tolerate the pressure of a sock or shoe.

At first, parents often refuse to believe this. They know their child loves the activities he or she is involved in. Any suggestion that there may be a psychological aspect to the problem is immediately rejected. Extensive experience with children with RSD, however, has allowed physicians to understand that it is invariably a cry for help. The key to solving the problem is for everyone involved to realize after careful investigation that it is not simply a physical injury. Once this is done, the child and family can concentrate on solving the related issues and working with their physicians and psychologists to fully resolve the problem. Physical therapy is often still necessary because of the long period of disuse.

DIAGNOSIS OF RSD

The first step in treating a child with RSD is to make sure the diagnosis is correct. While I have often seen physicians fail to make this diagnosis, I also have had children with undiagnosed arthritis referred as having RSD. In RSD, the blood work is usually normal. In long-standing cases, X-rays may show some mild osteoporosis due to disuse. An MRI may show some patchy marrow edema, and the bone scan may show increased uptake, decreased uptake, or patchy increased and decreased uptake.

On physical exam, the involved hand or foot is often markedly discolored. It may feel warm to the touch, but far more often it is cold. The child is often very tense when you examine the involved limb and may cry out with pain. However, it is often possible to distract or calmly reassure the child and proceed to examine the limb fully. Most often distraction or reassurance will not work if there is a fracture, infection, tumor, or other significant injury.

Making the diagnosis of RSD is usually far easier than explaining the diagnosis to the family and getting them to accept the diagnosis. Affected children are almost invariably overachievers who are very anxious to please their parents. In many cases, the combination of an abnormal bone scan and the obvious initial injury make it very difficult for the parents to accept the idea that there is a psychological issue.

RSD is a true somatization disorder. This means that the child really feels the pain, and the pain is real. The child is not making up a complaint of pain to manipulate the parents. Since the child is in pain and the injured extremity is discolored, parents ask, "How can this be psychological?" It takes a lot of explaining to make the family realize that you do not think this is something the child is making up. RSD is not a voluntary illness. A child does not say to herself, "If I say my foot hurts, I will not have to skate anymore." Whatever goes on in somatization disorders happens at a subconscious level that the child is no more aware of than the parents.

TREATMENT OF RSD

Once the diagnosis has been correctly made, physical therapy and psychological therapy become equally important. Physical therapy should concentrate on desensitization. The key is to persistently massage the tender extremity and gradually reassure the child that it is safe to put on a sock, to walk on the foot, or to use the hand. This is a process that may require weeks or months to accomplish. It should be accompanied by ongoing family psychological therapy to help the family and child understand the origins of the problem.

I have seen families refuse the psychological aspects of care and insist on only physical therapy. Although physical therapy may help even in the absence of psychological therapy, it fails to address the fact that this illness is a cry for help.

In several cases, children whose parents refused psychological intervention when I diagnosed RSD recovered from their chronic pain but ultimately required psychiatric hospitalization.

Parents of children with RSD should be aware that pain specialists often believe that drug therapy is appropriate for these children. Corticosteroids, regional sympathetic blocks, and narcotic analgesics all may provide temporary relief but fail to address the primary underlying problem. In several studies of large groups of children, it has been shown that the long-term outcome is far better for children treated with physical and psychological therapy than for children treated with medications and injections.

19

Osteoporosis and Osteopenia

Osteoporosis and osteopenia are conditions involving decreased bone mass and hence a decrease in the strength of the bones with an increased risk of fractures. Osteopenia has been defined as having bone mass that is more than one standard deviation below the normal level, and osteoporosis as having bone mass that is more than two and a half standard deviations below normal. These definitions have been difficult to apply to children because the normal levels have not been well defined for children of different ages and races. However, precise medical definitions are not what parents should be concerned about. What it is important for parents to understand is that children who do not get enough calcium in their diet, children with chronic arthritis, children who take corticosteroids or certain other drugs (especially diuretics such as furosemide), and children with a variety of hormonal disorders are all at risk of decreased bone mass and easily broken bones.

Decreased bone mass in children is particularly disturbing because bone mass normally increases during childhood and then begins to decrease during adult life. If a child never reaches his or her expected peak bone mass level as a young adult, the risk of having significant problems later in life, when everyone's bone mass normally decreases, is much greater than normal.

For parents, the first concern about osteoporosis or osteopenia may come when the doctor prescribes a medicine that is known to cause bone loss or when a doctor makes a casual comment when looking at the child's X-rays. Sometimes the osteoporosis is not noticed until the child complains of back pain due to vertebral fractures that are the result of osteoporosis.

If your child is taking anticonvulsants (medicines for seizures), diuretics (medicine to help kidney function), or corticosteroids, he or she should be monitored carefully. If a child is discovered to have osteoporosis or osteopenia and is not known to have arthritis or be taking medicines that cause the problem, he or she should be evaluated by an endocrinologist or bone specialist to determine the cause. Young female athletes who train extensively while eating poorly are at particular risk for osteoporosis and stress fractures. Teenagers should be specifically counseled that both alcohol and smoking increase the risk of osteoporosis.

While osteoporosis may be suspected on the basis of routine X-rays, bone density studies should be done to confirm the diagnosis using DEXA (dual energy X-ray absorptiometry) or a similar technique. It is important to use a method of measuring bone density that will provide quantitative results so that changes in bone density can be followed over time. There is no laboratory test to detect the problem, although there are tests that may help determine why a child has osteoporosis.

COMPLICATIONS OF OSTEOPOROSIS AND OSTEOPENIA

The major complications of osteoporosis are fractures of various kinds. Stress fractures in the limbs of athletes become evident as pain at the site of the fracture. Vertebral fractures in children with chronic disease cause severe back pain. Occasionally, children are recognized to have osteoporosis only when they fracture an arm or leg after a minor fall.

For children with an underlying rheumatic disease, the key to the prevention of osteoporosis is control of the inflammatory process. However, while corticosteroids are effective anti-inflammatory agents, they promote osteoporosis. They must be used very cautiously, but at the same time you do not want to risk serious damage from uncontrolled rheumatic disease because of the future risk of osteoporosis due to corticosteroids. Any child who must take corticosteroids needs to understand the importance of not taking extra when he or she feels bad. At times the doctor may find it necessary to increase the dose to improve disease control, but the doctor is also well aware of the need to reduce the dose as soon as the symptoms improve.

TREATMENT OF OSTEOPOROSIS AND OSTEOPENIA

The most important element of treatment for childhood osteoporosis is prevention. Every child should have an adequate calcium intake. If extra calcium is given in the form of supplements, it must be accompanied by vitamin D. However, while calcium and vitamin D are essential nutrients, excessive vitamin D consumption is dangerous and can even be fatal, and excessive intake of calcium should be avoided because it often causes constipation and stomach upset.

Attention to diet and appropriate supplementation should be adequate treatment for children with mild osteopenia. Children with fractures or DEXA-documented osteoporosis may require more aggressive therapy. However, appropriate treatment for children with osteoporosis remains controversial. Bisphosphonates such as alendronate and other drugs used in adults may be required. They prevent the withdrawal of calcium from bones and have been proven to reverse osteoporosis to some extent in children. However, their long-term safety for use in childhood is not established. Bisphosphonates are stored in the bones for many years. We do not know whether taking bisphosphonates earlier in life will cause problems for a woman if she becomes pregnant; this has limited our ability to use these drugs.

Calcitonin is an alternative therapy that deserves serious consideration. Calcitonin is a hormone that is normally made by the body to promote bone formation. Calcitonin isolated from fish is now available for prescription use. However, calcitonin is expensive and difficult to administer to children.

As noted above, the real key to successful treatment of osteoporosis is prevention. Monitoring the child's diet, emphasizing the negative effects of smoking and alcohol consumption on bone density, and whenever possible avoiding medications that cause osteoporosis are easily taken steps that should minimize the frequency of osteoporosis in childhood. In contrast, all of the drug regimens used to treat osteoporosis are of uncertain benefit if the cause of the osteoporosis has not been addressed.

PROGNOSIS FOR CHILDREN WITH OSTEOPOROSIS OR OSTEOPENIA

The prognosis for a child with osteopenia is very good. Identification of any underlying problem, correction of the diet, and appropriate medical therapy should lead to improvement. The prognosis for children with osteoporosis is more guarded. Parents must consider whether such children should be treated with bisphosphonates. Children with severe osteoporosis should be referred to large centers with experienced staff, where they can receive the best possible therapy.

PART III

LIVING WITH A CHILD WHO HAS A CHRONIC CONDITION

20

Medications and Immunizations

I want you to understand why your child should take medicine (if it has been prescribed) and how to be sure your child gets the best results. Understanding your child's medications and making sure he or she takes them appropriately are vitally important in getting the best outcome.

I do not discuss every possible medication in this chapter, just the medications I commonly use in the treatment of rheumatic disease; I do use others as the situation warrants. Different physicians have different approaches to medication use and different preferred medications. If your physician has recommended a medication not covered in this chapter, ask him or her for more information.

GENERAL CONCEPTS

Most parents are not happy about having to give their children medication on a long-term basis, and most children are not happy about having to take it. But children who do take their medicine routinely are the ones who get the best results.

Select a physician you trust and follow his or her instructions. The doctor will tell you about possible side effects of medications and will monitor your child appropriately. Appropriate monitoring, however, means that you must bring the child in for periodic visits and blood tests.

When to Withhold Your Child's Medication

This is a subject that is frequently overlooked. If your child is sick with the flu or a virus and not keeping anything down, you do not want to give him or her NSAIDs or immunosuppressive medications. The only arthritis medication that is vital to take even when one feels sick is corticosteroids (see below). All the other medications should be avoided, and you should call the doctor for instructions.

Children who are sick with a virus are also at risk of Reye's syndrome if they take certain medications. Reye's syndrome usually follows a viral infection and presents with symptoms of nausea, vomiting, and sleepiness. This is an unusual condition of uncertain cause. What is clear is that aspirin and other drugs, including NSAIDs such as ibuprofen (Motrin, Advil) and ibuprofen-containing products, may aggravate the condition. Untreated, Reye's syndrome can produce multiple complications that may be life-threatening.

It is also important not to give your child the medication if something goes wrong every time he or she takes it. If something unexpected is happening, it may be a side effect. The proper course of action is to stop giving the medication and call the doctor. If you keep giving the medication despite problems, you may make the whole situation worse. If you stop the medication because you think it's causing a side effect or not helping but do not tell the doctor, how is the doctor going to help you? If the medication the doctor has prescribed does not work for your child, call the doctor, who will prescribe a different one.

Getting Your Child to Take the Medication

Getting your child to take his or her medication depends a lot on the age of the child. For babies, all you can do with pills is mash them up and hide them in applesauce or another favorite food and make sure it goes down. Liquid medications can often be put in with formula. A compounding pharmacist can make many medications that do not come in liquid form into liquids, and add a flavor that the child likes. You may have to ask around to find one, and your insurance company may not always pay the cost, but it may be worthwhile just to avoid the aggravation. Each medication is different, so check with your doctor.

If your child is little, it's best to make taking medication a positive experience. However, remember to keep the medication well out of reach, as a small child who is rewarded for properly taking medication might take the whole bottle if he or she finds it. Liquid medicines may be combined with something that the child likes (chocolate milk is popular).

For small children, pills can sometimes be chewed or swallowed. Otherwise, they can be combined with foods that cover the texture and taste, such as chunky peanut butter. Smashed pills can also be put in the middle of cookies such as Oreos. Some parents have found it useful to break pills into pieces and slip them inside gelatinous candies such as gummy bears that have been cut partially open with a sharp knife.

Some pills are coated to make them easier to take or to delay their absorption. Crushing the pill interferes with the purpose of this coating, though sometimes there may be no alternative. However, certain pills are designed to release a controlled amount of medicine over time. These should not be crushed. If you are going to crush a pill, make sure you have discussed this with the doctor first.

For children over the age of six, education is important. They should understand when and why they take their medication, at least in broad general terms. Children over the age of twelve can usually be trusted to take their own medication, but there are always exceptions and you should base your judgment of this on your knowledge of your own child. Even if your child is a responsible teenager, you might ask yourself when the last time you had to refill the prescription was and how many pills are in the bottle. I've had disasters occur when children who were doing well for several years decided they really did not need their medicine anymore. By the time they realized they did need it and their parents and I discovered they were not taking it, it was too late to fix all the damage.

Children Who Fight Taking Their Medication

There are a number of elements to consider in dealing with children who fight taking their medication. The easiest answer is to avoid getting into this situation. Finding a suitable compromise by making the medication into a liquid or offering ice cream, candy, and so on is usually preferable to an all-out battle. For children in the younger age groups, a reward system (or bribery) is often the easiest and most effective answer. As parents, we all believe that we should not have to bribe our children to get them to do what they should be doing anyway. However, over years of watching parents deal with their children, it's become clear to me that whether it's called a reward system or bribery, giving your children positive reinforcement for taking their medication works better than anything else.

If there are continuing problems in getting the child to take medication, it is important to deal with them openly. As children grow up they become increasingly frustrated by their lack of control over what happens to them. Often a struggle over taking medication is really a statement that says, "I hate having my disease." If everyone can sit down and discuss what's going on, it may be possible to simply talk it out. If not, psychological intervention may be required. Often a child who completely refuses to take medication will respond quickly to being placed in a hospital environment where nurses instead of parents administer the medication. Awareness that the medication is a symbol of the disease and may become a focus of normal parent-child conflicts may help everyone bring the situation to a quick resolution.

What if the Medicine Is Not Working?

This question has no simple answer. It depends on the type of medication and the disease. Your child might have been given the wrong medicine. Call your doctor and make sure the name of the medication on the bottle is what it is supposed to be. Not every doctor writes clearly and not every pharmacist reads carefully.

Most medications have a trade name and a generic name. Your doctor might have called the medication by its trade name and it may be labeled with the generic name. If you are unsure, check. Today the trade and generic names of drugs can be found on the Internet in just a few minutes. If you don't have easy access to the Internet, take a few minutes to call your doctor's office and have someone check that your child is taking the correct medication.

If your child is taking the drug your physician recommended and it is not working, you might be expecting results too quickly. Some arthritis medicines do not make a big difference until they have been taken for several weeks. Other medicines may be very important, but instead of making the child feel better, they prevent him or her from getting worse. Be sure you talk to your doctor about your concerns. If you are not comfortable talking with your doctor or the office staff, you need to find a doctor you can be comfortable talking with.

Generic medications are another area of concern. Not all generic medications are equally effective. Some manufacturers make very good generics that can save you money. Others, however, have less stringent quality controls. When you get a generic medicine from your pharmacist, you have to look carefully at the label to determine who made it. If you have been taking a generic made by one manufacturer without difficulty and then have problems, check to see whether the pharmacy gave you pills from another manufacturer. Even though the amount of drug in each pill may be the same, the coatings to prevent stomach problems, the ease with which the pill dissolves, and the filler material in the pill may all be entirely different. I have had patients suddenly get worse when they were changed to a generic. However, I also had a patient who got worse when he was changed from the generic to the brand-name pills.

Proper Monitoring

In this section I discuss the monitoring procedures that I believe should be done to get the best possible results. Keep in mind that this may not reflect every doctor's standard of care.

Medicines tend to have two types of side effects. The first is an idiosyncratic reaction, in which the patient responds to the drug in an unusual way. This is similar to an allergic reaction but not usually a true allergy. Some people are just unusually sensitive to certain medicines. The other type of side effect is related to the amount of the medicine, in terms of both the amount taken in each dose and the total amount taken over time. These side effects require different types of monitoring.

For medicines such as NSAIDs, which are generally safe, I want children to be tested within two or three weeks of starting the medicine to look for any unusual reactions, six weeks after starting the medicine to look for any cumulative reactions, three months after starting the medicine, and then every three months thereafter. This is very conservative, careful monitoring, but as a result I have never encountered a serious medication side effect that did not resolve. There are many physicians who check much less frequently; usually there is no problem.

For medicines that are known to have an increased frequency or severity of side effects, such as methotrexate, I ask my patients to get their blood checked every week at the beginning, then every two weeks. Only when I am sure they are tolerating the medicine well at the full dose do I extend the frequency of blood tests to every month and eventually every three months. If parents add a new supplement to the child's diet, I start the monitoring tests over again, as some supplements have side effects, either by themselves or in combination with certain medications. I recommend that children on supplements be monitored just as carefully as children on prescription medicines. There are numerous well-documented cases of children who became ill from dietary supplements.

Why Take Medicines if They Are Potentially Dangerous?

It can be difficult for a parent to give a child medication that carries the risk of serious side effects. However, if the benefits of these drugs did not far outweigh the risks, no physician would be recommending them. And most medicines are not normally dangerous.

In cases where a child's medical condition is life-threatening, the choice of whether to give a medication that potentially has serious side effects is usually not difficult. But parents may be more reluctant if the problem seems to be only a sore knee. However, if it is not controlled with medication, the underlying condition causing that sore knee may eventually cause far more significant damage to joints, bones, and organs that may go unnoticed until it has become irreversible and will dramatically affect the child's health and quality of life in the future.

What about situations where the medication is simply making the child feel better, not altering the course of the disease? The first thing to remember when dealing with children with arthritis or any other disease is that we want the best possible outcome in terms of ability to function, not just day to day but in later adult life as well. If children's medical problems are interfering with their ability to keep up with their friends and do normal things, it's interfering with their concept of who they are and their feelings of self-worth. Failure to take care of these problems may have disastrous consequences in both the short and long terms.

Why Continue to Take Medication Even After the Child Feels Better?

Many of the diseases I treat are chronic and recurrent. They can be controlled, but they can never be pronounced gone. When the disease is under control, the parents and their children would like to forget about it. I've seen children suffer permanent damage because their parents thought the problem was gone, stopped the medicines, and stopped coming for checkups and blood work. The doctor will tell you if it seems possible to stop the medication. Until then, it is extremely important to keep taking the medication.

NONSTEROIDAL ANTI-INFLAMMATORY DRUGS

Nonsteroidal anti-inflammatory drugs (NSAIDs) are the mainstay of therapy for most children with rheumatic disease. All of them interfere to varying degrees with the cyclooxygenase pathway, which is responsible for the production of prostaglandins, important inflammatory mediators (chemicals that cause fever, pain, and irritation). By blocking the production of these inflammatory mediators, NSAIDs serve to reduce the amount of pain, fever, and irritation that the child experiences. Most of the NSAIDs interfere with the chemicals cyclooxygenase-1 (COX-1) and cyclooxygenase-2 (COX-2). Choosing the proper NSAID for a given child involves balancing convenience, cost, effectiveness, and probability of side effects.

Side Effects of NSAIDs

Allergic reactions can occur with any medications. Few children are allergic to NSAIDs, but if there is a history of allergy to aspirin or similar medications, caution is warranted. Some children who are allergic to aspirin are allergic to all

NSAIDs, but others are not. You will need to work carefully with your doctor to evaluate this problem if it occurs.

All NSAIDs may irritate the lining of the stomach. This may cause indigestion or loss of appetite. It is important to make sure the child takes the medicine on a full stomach. If the stomachaches are common or persistent, make sure your doctor is aware. He or she may choose to change the medication or add another medication to protect the stomach lining. Some children have developed ulcers while taking NSAIDs, but this is uncommon. Remember, if every NSAID causes a child to have stomachaches, perhaps something else is going on.

Bruising is a common side effect of all of the COX-1 NSAIDs. These drugs interfere with platelet stickiness and cause the child to bleed or bruise more than he or she would otherwise. Frequent bruises over the shins are common for children on NSAIDs, but if they are significant, the physician should do blood tests to make sure there is not another explanation. It is also important to stop the NSAIDs before any elective surgery where there is a high risk of bleeding. Consult the physician doing the surgery. It may be necessary to stop the NSAIDs two weeks in advance.

Liver irritation may also occur with these medications. Most often the patient is not aware of the liver irritation and it is detected only by blood work. With aspirin, liver irritation was very common and mild inflammation of the liver was tolerated. Given the variety of medications available today, we are less tolerant of liver irritation, but minimal amounts are acceptable.

The NSAIDs also affect the kidneys. They usually interfere with the rate at which the kidneys filter the blood. This means that the child will hold more water in the body. This causes a few pounds of weight gain and may be reflected in a drop in the hemoglobin value and slight rise in the BUN level. These are normal effects of the medications.

In some children using NSAIDs, the kidneys become irritated, resulting in a condition called interstitial nephritis. This is a more serious condition that requires stopping the NSAID. It may have to be treated with steroids and could result in permanent damage. Routine urine tests are part of monitoring for side effects of NSAIDs in order to detect any signs of this problem. It may not occur until many months or years after starting the medication. This is why the monitoring must continue.

An unusual skin rash called a pseudoporphyria reaction has been described in some children on NSAIDs. This skin rash appears when the child is out in the sun. At first, it just looks like a number of tiny blisters. However, the blisters leave a small scar when they heal. With continued medication and continued sun exposure, there will be more and more blisters and scars. The medication should be stopped and the sun avoided until the medicine is cleared from the body. This reaction has been noticed most often with naproxen, but that may be because so much naproxen is used. It has been reported with other NSAIDs, and all children on NSAIDs should be monitored for it.

Behavioral problems in children taking chronic medication can result from many different causes. In general, the NSAIDs do *not* cause misbehavior, changes in attitude, poor sleeping, difficulty studying, or similar side effects. However, very strong NSAIDs, such as indomethacin, are known to cause headaches, depression, and dizziness. If there is a significant behavioral problem in a child on an NSAID, I will observe at first and then stop or change the NSAID to see whether there is an improvement in the problem.

This list is not comprehensive, and other problems may occur. If you are concerned that your child may be experiencing a side effect of medication, be sure to discuss it with your doctor.

Choosing the Correct NSAID

As a physician, I want to give children with arthritis the NSAID that makes them better with the least likelihood of side effects and the greatest convenience. Like most doctors, I start with the easy ones and carefully move on to the stronger ones if the response to the easy ones is inadequate. The list of side effects is essentially the same for all the NSAIDs; it is the probability of the side effects that changes.

One of the most common problems is for children to be treated with only one NSAID and told there is no other choice. The physician may either stick with that NSAID even though it is not working well or recommend jumping to a second-line drug without trying any other NSAID. Despite their similar mechanisms of action, all NSAIDs are not the same. Some of the NSAIDs are far more effective for certain types of arthritis. Failure to recognize the different types of juvenile arthritis (see Chapter 5) means that many doctors do not realize that different NSAIDs are better for different types of diseases.

Many physicians will not prescribe NSAIDs that have not been specifically tested and approved by the Food and Drug Administration (FDA) for use in children. However, the testing costs a lot of money and there are not that many children with arthritis. As a result, many excellent drugs have never been specifically approved for children. That does not mean that they cannot or should not be used by physicians who are experienced with them, do appropriate monitoring, and are comfortable with their use. In some cases, newer drugs have been shown to be more effective and safer, but some physicians continue to use the less effective and more toxic drugs in children because no one has specifically told them the safer drug is approved for children. Changing to the appropriate NSAID can often make a dramatic difference for a child. However, it may take some trial and error.

In what follows I discuss the NSAIDs that are commonly used and the ones I prefer to use. This is not a complete list of all NSAIDs or of every NSAID I ever use. I have found a variety of NSAIDs that I am comfortable using in children and feel are effective. I have not tried them all, and the absence of an NSAID from this list simply means I do not use it often. A few, like aspirin, are included because other physicians commonly use them, even though I rarely do. The FDA has not specifically approved all of these medications for use in children at this time. That means they cannot be advertised "for use by children"; however, it does not mean children cannot use them.

Aspirin

Aspirin was the original NSAID and was the mainstay of therapy when I began my career. On a worldwide basis aspirin remains one of the most widely used treatments for children with arthritis. However, its use in the United States is limited by the ready availability of other medications that are more convenient, equally effective, and less likely to cause side effects. It has disadvantages: it needs to be given three or four times a day, it is available only as pills, and it frequently upsets the stomach.

Although aspirin is available without a prescription, regular use must be monitored, just like the use of prescription NSAIDs, to minimize the risk of severe and even life-threatening side effects. An additional concern in the use of aspirin is that it has been linked to Reye's syndrome (discussed above).

Naproxen and Ibuprofen

Naproxen (marketed as Aleve and Naprosyn, among other brand names) and ibuprofen (Motrin, Advil, Nuprin) are available in liquid form and are used extensively in the treatment of children with arthritis. Naproxen has an advantage in being given twice a day, while ibuprofen may need to be given as many as four times a day. Ibuprofen liquid and pills, and some forms of naproxen pills, are available without a prescription. The reason ibuprofen liquid is available without prescription while naproxen liquid is not is unclear. Both of these drugs require monitoring, just like all the other NSAIDs, whether a doctor prescribes them or you buy them without a prescription. Other than stomach upset, side effects of these medications are relatively infrequent. However, all of the side effects listed in the section on NSAID side effects may occur. These NSAIDs are effective for true pauciarticular-onset JA and helpful in many other conditions. For many children with more difficult forms of JA, more potent NSAIDs may be necessary.

Nabumetone

Nabumetone (marketed as Relafen) seems to be very effective for arthritis while rarely causing stomach irritation. It's easy for parents because it has to be given only once each day. Although it does not come as a liquid, it will dissolve in warm water without any apparent loss in efficacy. It can also be crushed. Since it has a long half-life (it stays in the body longer, which is why it needs to be given only once a day), it can easily be given after dinner for a peak effect the next morning, when it helps to reduce morning stiffness.

Diclofenac and Tolmetin Sodium

Diclofenac and tolmetin sodium are marketed as Voltaren and Tolectin, respectively. They are effective for all onset types of JA and for spondyloarthropathies. Many children who are not doing well enough on naproxen or ibuprofen dramatically improve when switched to diclofenac. However, complaints of stomachache and increases in liver enzymes seem more common with these medications. Physicians prescribing them must monitor the children for these problems. In general, I prefer diclofenac to tolmetin because of fewer complaints of stomach irritation; also most preparations of diclofenac (except the liquid form for small children, which must be prepared by a compounding pharmacist) are enteric-coated to protect the stomach.

Piroxicam

Piroxicam (marketed as Feldene) is an NSAID that is very effective for many older children with spondyloarthropathies and the related types of arthritis.

It has a very long half-life and slowly builds up to an effective level in the body. Often it takes two or three weeks to start having an effect. However, it is frequently very effective when other NSAIDs have not been sufficient. Gastrointestinal side effects and renal side effects may be more common with piroxicam than with other NSAIDs and do not always occur at the beginning of therapy.

Indomethacin

Indomethacin (marketed as Indocin) is generally agreed to be the most potent of the routinely used NSAIDs. It is an excellent inhibitor of inflammation. Indomethacin is also much more likely to cause side effects. In addition to the side effects listed for all NSAIDs, it is common for children on indomethacin to complain of headaches. However, many of the children old enough to talk about it say that the trade-off in improved relief of arthritis is worthwhile. The headaches can be treated with acetaminophen and do decrease in frequency and severity over time. Some individuals become depressed when taking indomethacin, and the physician and family must watch out for this complication. In small children, it may cause inexplicable temper tantrums. Kidney and liver irritation are also well-recognized side effects. Indomethacin is available as a liquid.

In children with systemic-onset arthritis, indomethacin may relieve fever and other symptoms when no other NSAID is effective. Indomethacin is also very effective for some children with spondyloarthropathies who have not responded to other NSAIDs. However, it requires careful monitoring. Chemically, diclofenac and nabumetone are more closely related to indomethacin than most others. They are not as strong as indomethacin, but significant side effects occur far less often.

Celecoxib

Celecoxib (marketed as Celebrex) is a useful NSAID that provides a good level of relief for some children. Celecoxib is available as a liquid and has been specifically approved for children. It has a reduced frequency of side effects, but this medication does contain sulfa, and children who are allergic to sulfa drugs may be allergic to celecoxib.

There has been a lot of concern about the incidence of heart attacks in people taking COX-2 inhibitors, some of which were pulled off the market because of this. However, no pediatric rheumatologist ever reported a child with a heart attack on these drugs, and it is important to remember that no drug is ever completely safe.

Sucralfate

This drug is not an anti-inflammatory, but I include sucralfate (sold as Carafate) under this category because it was developed to minimize stomach irritation secondary to other medications. It is frequently added by rheumatologists if a child complains of stomach irritation with NSAIDs. It essentially coats the stomach but lets the medicine get absorbed into the body.

The key thing to remember about sucralfate is that it takes time for the medication to dissolve in the stomach and spread over the surface to provide its protective action. The child should take the sucralfate at least a half an hour in advance of the other medicines. If the medicines is taken with meals, give the child the sucralfate before the meal and the others immediately after the meal.

Side effects of sucralfate are rare. A few people have been allergic to it. Others have complained of bloating or constipation. Some of my patients say it makes them feel full. It is available in liquid form for small children.

OTHER DRUGS WITH ANTI-INFLAMMATORY ACTION

Sulfasalazine

Sulfasalazine (Azulfidine), which combines salicylic acid (a precursor of aspirin) with sulfapyridine (an antibiotic), is an older drug that is very effective for spondyloarthropathies, especially in children who have not responded to other NSAIDs, but less effective for other forms of arthritis in childhood. Its mechanism of action is unclear. Sulfasalazine can be used in addition to other NSAIDs.

The major disadvantage of sulfasalazine is that anyone who is allergic to sulfa drugs will be to be allergic to sulfasalazine. These allergies often take the form of skin rashes that can be quite dramatic. Other common side effects include liver irritation, stomach upset, and decreased white blood cell count. Allergic reactions require stopping the drug; other problems might respond to changing the dose. Because of the allergic reactions, I usually start children on a small dose of sulfasalazine and monitor them carefully as I increase the dose.

If a child does not have an allergic reaction to the drug, he or she can often tolerate it without difficulty for years, properly monitored. I have many patients who did not need to take potentially more toxic medications such as methotrexate because this drug was effective for them.

Hydroxychloroquine

Hydroxychloroquine (brand name Plaquenil) is a derivative of quinine, which was originally used to fight malaria. Quinine was first reported to be beneficial for patients with rheumatic disease in the 1890s; hydroxychloroquine is a derivative that has fewer side effects. The precise mechanism of action of hydroxychloroquine remains unknown. The drug is very slow in its onset of action—the child will not take one and feel better immediately—but many controlled studies have shown that the group of patients receiving hydroxychloroquine did better than the group that did not.

Hydroxychloroquine has been found to be helpful in children with most forms of arthritis, systemic lupus erythematosus, dermatomyositis, and scleroderma in both its localized and systemic forms. It is probably helpful for many other conditions as well. At one time, it was thought that hydroxychloroquine was uniquely effective for skin manifestations of dermatomyositis and SLE, but it is not clear that this is true.

One of the most interesting things about hydroxychloroquine is that evidence suggests that it can change the long-term outcome of the disease rather than just relieve symptoms. It is rarely associated with toxicity. Although some listings of potential side effects include blindness, it is important to know that this warning comes from a period in the late 1960s and early 1970s when the wrong dosage was used. Once the dosage was corrected, this problem essentially disappeared. Your physician will recommend an eye examination by an ophthalmologist before your child starts the drug and every six months while taking the drug. This is to check for any evidence of damage to the eye by the hydroxychloroquine.

Checking the child's eyes before starting the medication allows the physicians to detect any abnormality that might be present for another reason. If this was not noted before starting and found while the child was taking hydroxychloroquine, it might be mistakenly thought to have come from the hydroxychloroquine. In many years of prescribing hydroxychloroquine, I have had a small number of patients where the ophthalmologist thought there might be an early problem and I stopped the medication. I have never had a child or parent notice any vision-related problem due to hydroxychloroquine.

Since hydroxychloroquine appears to be safe and effective but very slow-acting, children are often kept on it for years. Like all medications, hydroxychloroquine can be associated with a wide variety of minor complaints or abnormalities on blood tests and so needs to be monitored appropriately. Fortunately, these problems are very infrequent. Hydroxychloroquine is unique in that it is probably one of the worst-tasting pills. The modern preparation is coated so that it can be swallowed without being tasted, but if you have to crush or break the pill for your child, it tastes terrible. A compounding pharmacist can provide it in liquid form and add ingredients to hide the taste.

Doxycycline

Doxycycline is marketed under a wide variety of trade names around the world, including Vibramycin. It is a tetracycline antibiotic that is also useful for patients with arthritis. The use of doxycycline and related tetracyclines in children is restricted by the fact that tetracyclines permanently stain growing teeth. Most physicians prefer not to use doxycycline before the age of ten, though some will use it earlier.

It has been shown that doxycycline works in arthritis by blocking a group of enzymes called metalloproteinases. This effect is independent of its effect as an antibiotic. Chemists were able to synthesize a derivative of doxycycline that did not work as an antibiotic but still reduced arthritis.

In addition to staining teeth in young children, doxycycline causes a number of children to complain of stomach upset and photosensitivity (they burn easily in the sun). These complaints limit its use as well. It is also used in the treatment of acne in teenagers and in the treatment of Lyme disease. Some caution using doxycycline for acne is necessary, because it has been associated with rare cases of drug-induced SLE.

There are a number of good controlled studies indicating that doxycycline is an effective adjunctive (extra) agent for patients with arthritis, but the vast majority of teenagers I give it to discontinue it because of chronic stomachaches. Patients also must be warned that they should always use sunblock and be careful when exposed to the sun for prolonged periods.

IMMUNOSUPPRESSIVE DRUGS

If a child with arthritis has failed to respond to NSAIDs, hydroxychloroquine, and sulfasalazine, the family will have to consider immunosuppressive medications or one of the newer biologics discussed below (although the biologics are classified separately, they are in fact immunosuppressive). The majority of children with arthritis do not require immunosuppressive drugs, but children with more severe arthritis will do much better if they are appropriately treated and their disease is brought under good control. Stronger immunosuppressive drugs are commonly used for children with illnesses such as systemic lupus erythematosus, dermatomyositis, scleroderma, polyarteritis nodosa, and Wegener's granulomatosis.

There are several important considerations in the use of immunosuppressive drugs for arthritis and related conditions. In the high dosages used for the treatment of children with cancer, these drugs have many major side effects. However, in general the dosage of the immunosuppressive drugs used in the treatment of children with arthritis is far lower, and so the risk of side effects drops.

I must repeat here that over my thirty years of caring for children with rheumatic diseases, the majority of the poor outcomes I have seen were the result of families refusing aggressive therapy for severe disease. If your doctor is recommending aggressive therapy, it is because the doctor believes it is more likely that your child will suffer permanent injury from the disease than from the medication. With careful monitoring, poor outcomes due to medication are extremely rare.

Certain potential side effects do have to be considered with every immunosuppressive medication. The two most important are the increased risk of infection and the possible increased risk of a malignancy (cancer) later in life.

In all of the rheumatic diseases, the body is acting as if it is trying to control an infection. The inflammatory reactions that result involve the release of many damaging substances (cytokines and similar agents) that are intended to kill bacteria and viruses but which in fact wind up damaging the joints and other tissues. Immunosuppressive drugs block the production of these damaging substances, thus preventing the damage to the joints and other tissues.

Some immunosuppressive drugs (such as cyclosporine, tacrolimus, etanercept, infliximab, adalimumab, and anakinra) work by directly blocking the messengers that stimulate production of the damaging substances. Other immunosuppressive drugs (rituximab and abatacept) work by interfering with the synthesis of inflammatory mediators or the cells that are stimulating the response. However, if a child on immunosuppressive drugs develops an infection, he or she does not have full use of these substances to fight off the infection. This is why careful monitoring and an experienced physician are so important.

In addition to preventing infections, the immune system is charged with monitoring the body for any cells that have reproduced themselves incorrectly (e.g., something goes wrong when the DNA is being copied). If the immune system finds a cell that is incorrectly made, it tries to destroy it. Some incorrectly made cells are the beginnings of cancer. Because the immunosuppressive drugs weaken the immune system, it might be easier for some of these cells to escape detection and become cancer. Moreover, the drugs that interfere with DNA synthesis may fail to kill a cell and instead cause it to develop incorrectly.

So why would anybody ever take immunosuppressive drugs? Again, it's a matter of balance. Physicians reserve these drugs for children whom they expect will do poorly if they are not aggressively treated. Every immunosuppressive drug increases the risk of infection. Every immunosuppressive drug increases the risk of having cancer later in life. Every immunosuppressive drug may interfere with the ability to have children. But at the dosages normally used for the treatment of children with arthritis, all of these problems are rare. Most often immunosuppressive drugs simply make you better.

Methotrexate

Methotrexate has significantly improved the outlook for many children with arthritis. As noted above, much of what you may read about negative effects of methotrexate is related to the doses used in the treatment of children with cancer, which are frequently tens or in some cases hundreds of times higher than the doses used to treat arthritis.

In the doses used in cancer therapy, methotrexate works by interfering with DNA synthesis and blocking the rapid reproduction of cells. However, in the dosage normally used for children with arthritis, methotrexate is believed to have a different mechanism of action. Nonetheless, it is very effective at reducing pain and swelling for children with most forms of arthritis. Careful studies in adults suggest that it may actually modify the course of the disease, and it certainly improves function and controls arthritis symptoms for most children who take it.

Most often methotrexate is given as pills (or shots) that are taken just once each week. Some physicians start out at the full dose and monitor blood work after a few weeks. However, there are children who are unexpectedly sensitive to methotrexate. I prefer to start out with a small dose and monitor the blood tests every week until I am sure the child is tolerating the drug. Children on methotrexate should take folic acid, which has sharply reduced the frequency of side effects. My patients take 1 mg every day (even the day when they take the methotrexate) and do fine.

At higher doses, many physicians prefer to give methotrexate as an injection. This has the advantage of consistently delivering the same dose to the body. If a child is taking pills, he or she may not get the same effect every week because of differences in what was eaten the day the pills were taken and other factors that influence the absorption of the methotrexate from the stomach. In addition, methotrexate injected under the skin is absorbed and distributed through the circulation before it reaches the liver, whereas pills are digested and go into the blood vessels that go directly to the liver. Since methotrexate is known to have a negative effect on the liver, at higher doses it is thought the shots are safer.

The onset of action of methotrexate is slow. It usually begins to show effects after a few weeks, but it may be six to twelve weeks before it is clearly having a significant effect on the arthritis. This is especially true if it is begun carefully, using a low dosage. For many children, methotrexate is a very effective drug and provides excellent control of the arthritis.

Many children who were having significant problems with arthritis do well after starting on methotrexate. Although there is no uniform agreement, most physicians will keep children on methotrexate until they have been well for at least six months. Some physicians then reduce the weekly dose, while others prefer to spread the dose out so that it is given every two weeks, then every three weeks, and so on, until it is slowly discontinued over a period of many months. Unfortunately, the arthritis flares in a substantial proportion of children as the methotrexate is withdrawn.

Common side effects of methotrexate include nausea, minor changes in the white blood cell or platelet count, and liver irritation. The nausea often responds to reassurance, but if it is severe, it can be treated with ondansetron (Zofran). Changes in the blood counts and liver enzymes are monitored through the blood work. Sores in the mouth or an irritated tongue may occur but are rare in children also taking folic acid. Children with warts will often notice that their warts either return or get worse when the methotrexate reaches an effective level.

Children taking methotrexate also need to be careful about going out in the sun. Although most children have no problem, some children are very easily sunburned when they are on methotrexate. It is important to be sure that your child is not excessively photosensitive before spending a day in the sun when he or she is on methotrexate. Another side effect of methotrexate noted in adults is rapid appearance of rheumatoid nodules during methotrexate therapy. This is rare in children.

In addition to the side effects discussed for immunosuppressive drugs in general, methotrexate may have side effects that include problems with the blood cell counts or liver function. In rare cases, methotrexate can also cause kidney and lung problems. It should be very carefully monitored in children with pre-existing liver, kidney, or lung conditions. Methotrexate is normally excreted by the kidneys, but it is not removed by dialysis. If your child has serious kidney problems, make sure your doctor is aware.

Children with persistent or recurrent liver enzyme abnormalities should be taken off methotrexate. Failure to do so could result in long-term liver damage. However, this is rarely necessary.

Occasional mild abnormalities in the white blood cell count or liver enzymes may be the result of viral infections or other unrelated problems. These situations are best dealt with by withholding the methotrexate until the problem corrects itself, then restarting the methotrexate while monitoring carefully to make sure the problem does not return. Everyone must remember that individuals using methotrexate must not drink alcoholic beverages, as the use of alcohol greatly increases the risk of liver damage. If your child drinks alcohol, make sure the doctor knows. If you can't trust the child to stop drinking, don't let him or her take methotrexate.

BIOLOGICS

The biologics are a new class of medications that have allowed us to provide dramatic relief to children with severe arthritis. Each is designed to target a specific molecule that plays an important role in the inflammatory process. Because the biologics relieve arthritis by directly affecting the immune response, they are immunosuppressive. As a result, the biologics carry the same risks of infection and possibly later development of cancer that are discussed in the section on immunosuppressive medications, above. Although in the past methotrexate was commonly prescribed before biologics, it has a slower onset of action, is often less effective, and has a higher frequency of side effects involving the bone marrow and liver. As a result, many physicians are moving to biologics before methotrexate. The biologics are more expensive, but in the long run their early use appears cost-effective. For the most severe cases it has shown that biologics and methotrexate are synergistic, and it may be necessary to add methotrexate after starting a biologic if it has not been used before.

Parents often worry that because the biologics are new medications, we do not know what will happen to someone who takes them for long periods. It's true that until a medication has been in use for a number of years, it will be impossible to know for sure what effects it will have. But all medications licensed for use in the United States have undergone several years of testing in animals and patients before they were licensed. Before you insist that you have to know what the effects of ten years of the medication might be before you allow your child to take it, remember that pediatric rheumatologists know quite well what ten years of uncontrolled arthritis will do to your child. There are remote risks of undiscovered long-term medication side effects, but we recommend these medicines because we know for sure that ten years of uncontrolled arthritis will cause significant disability.

It is recommended that any child at risk for tuberculosis be appropriately screened before beginning any biologic agent because of the drugs' immunosuppressive activity.

TNF Inhibitors

There are a variety of biologic agents currently available which interfere with the activity of tumor necrosis factor alpha (TNF-α), and several more are in early clinical testing. When large amounts of TNF-α are in the circulation, people tend to feel very ill. The effects of blocking TNF-α are often very impressive. Parents frequently report striking improvement within hours of the first dose. For most children, the improvement continues for as long as the child remains on a TNF inhibitor. These medications not only prevent symptoms of the disease but also allow healing of the bone and joint damage to begin.

Common side effects of TNF inhibitors include runny nose, injection site reactions, and headaches. Few parents or children feel these are significant when measured against the dramatic relief of arthritis symptoms. Periodic monitoring via blood tests is required, as with every medication, but significant problems are few.

There are several important considerations regarding uncommon side effects for children on TNF inhibitors. The most important is the increased risk of infection. Fortunately, serious infections are rare. Because of the risk of severe infections, if a child receiving TNF inhibitors looks sick, he or she should be seen by a doctor sooner, not later. In this situation I err on the side of antibiotic coverage.

TNF inhibitors and other biologics should not be given to children with fevers unless the fever is part of the disease they are being treated for (and then only with care). Skin and lung infections may be the most important to watch for. Infection is a risk with all of the immunosuppressive medications used for children with severe arthritis.

Another concern is that all of the drugs that affect the immune system may lead to the development or worsening of other diseases. Some children receiving TNF inhibitors have developed minor serologic abnormalities related to lupus, and this needs to be monitored. However, medically significant problems appear to be extremely rare. For the majority of children, allowing the arthritis to continue is far more dangerous than the remote risk of a serious side effect from TNF inhibitors.

Parents often ask how long their child will need to continue on TNF inhibitors. This is a very difficult question to answer. Although these medications do an excellent job of controlling disease, they do not cure it. I have had two experiences with children who seemed cured by TNF inhibitors, so much so that the family thought there was no reason to continue the shots or return for their appointments. After six or eight weeks off medication, however, the disease came back much worse than before.

Parents often become so worried after hearing about all the potential side effects that they hesitate about starting TNF inhibitors. You should know that the most common thing I hear from parents after they start children on these medications is "She's doing wonderfully. Why did you let me wait so long?"

At the present time, a child who is doing well on TNF inhibitors should continue on the medication. After a year of doing well it is often possible to decrease the frequency of injections. The proper means of discontinuing TNF inhibitors remains to be determined. In the few children for whom TNF inhibitors has not been beneficial, there have been no problems with discontinuing it.

Etanercept

Etanercept (sold as Enbrel) was the first widely available biologic. The etanercept molecule consists of two artificial receptors for TNF-α attached to an Fc receptor that allows the etanercept to which TNF has bound to be cleared from the body. It has made a dramatic difference in the care of children with JA.

Many pediatric rheumatologists feel it is the most significant advance in many years. It is effective for most children with polyarticular-onset arthritis, spondyloarthropathies, and psoriatic arthritis and some children with systemic-onset arthritis. It may prove to be effective for many other forms of childhood rheumatic disease, but this has not been fully investigated. Although etanercept is also effective for children with severe pauciarticular-onset arthritis, it is infrequently necessary for that disease.

Etanercept was initially studied in children with severe disease who were not responding adequately to methotrexate. All of the data that have been published indicate that methotrexate plus etanercept is better than methotrexate alone. However, etanercept is now commonly used alone because of the lower frequency of side effects. Many physicians add methotrexate only in more difficult cases that have not responded to etanercept or another biologic. The major disadvantage of etanercept is that it must be given by subcutaneous injection weekly. The shots can be given in the physician's office or at home by a visiting nurse or another individual. However, since subcutaneous injections are easy to do, most parents learn to do them without difficulty.

Common side effects of etanercept include runny nose, injection site reactions, and headaches. Uncommon side effects are listed in the general section on TNF inhibitors, above.

Adalimumab

This is another of the new of the biologics. Adalimumab (trade name Humira) is an antibody to TNF-α that can be given as a subcutaneous injection either every week or every other week. Not only does it attack TNF-α in the circulation, but it can also attack TNF-α molecules on the surface of cells, destroying both the TNF-α and the cells. It is a very effective treatment for severe arthritis. It works well for most children with polyarticular-onset arthritis, spondyloarthropathies, and psoriatic arthritis and some children with systemic-onset arthritis. It may also prove to be effective for many other forms of childhood arthritis.

Adalimumab has been effective in some children who have not responded to etanercept. In addition, Adalimumab has been an extremely effective agent in the treatment of children with uveitis associated with arthritis. Because adalimumab is what's called a fully humanized antibody (that is, it has been modified to appear to the immune system as if it were made in the body), there appear to be fewer side effects, and the body's immune system is less likely to produce human antichimeric antibodies (HACAs) that attack the adalimumab molecule and block its effect than is the case with infliximab. Adalimumab has also proven effective in the treatment of Crohn's disease and seems particularly effective in children with psoriatic arthritis. Although adalimumab acts by directly binding to TNF-α rather than being a "fake receptor," because it also serves to block the activity of TNF-α it shares with etanercept the increased risk of infection and possible future development of malignancy. Adalimumab and etanercept have a similar frequency of side effects, but adalimumab requires less frequent injections that etanercept. Children receiving adalimumab should be cautioned that the injections sting; children who know to expect this seem to tolerate them without difficulty. The efficacy of adalimumab in children who have conditions that do not respond well to etanercept is sufficient to offset the discomfort of its use.

It should be noted that the official product literature for adalimumab suggests that the injections be given every other week and increased to weekly only if the drug has proven ineffective. I often find it more effective to give adalimumab weekly for the first six to twelve weeks and establish good control of the inflammation, then decrease the frequency of injections. For children with uveitis, weekly injections often needed to be continued indefinitely.

Infliximab

Infliximab (Remicade) is another antibody that is directed against TNF-α. In the published information on infliximab, it is suggested for use in conjunction with methotrexate. This is because, as with adalimumab, the antibody molecule that is the active part of infliximab sometimes stimulates an immune response in which the body produces human antichimeric antibodies, which attack the infliximab molecule and block its effect. There is reason to believe that taking methotrexate slows the formation of HACAs. It is also believed that methotrexate reduces the incidence of allergic reactions and other complications that may interfere with how infliximab works. If a child cannot tolerate methotrexate and requires infliximab, it may be useful to treat him or her with one of the other immunosuppressive drugs.

The major difficulties associated with infliximab relate to its administration. Infliximab is given as a periodic intravenous infusion. It can be given in a physician's office, in a hospital infusion unit, or by a visiting nurse. The dosage regimen is variable. After the initial doses, which are given more frequently, infliximab may be given monthly or every other month. The optimal dosage regimen and frequency are not the same for every patient. Allergic reactions seem to be more common with infliximab than other biologics, and some patients need to be medicated for these. As a result, the first dose of infliximab is normally given under a doctor's supervision. Even after the first dose, any side effects during administration should be promptly reported to the physician for evaluation.

Infection is a concern with infliximab, just as it is with other immunosuppressive and biologic agents. Tuberculosis is a particular concern, and children should be screened for tuberculosis and tuberculosis exposure before infliximab is begun. The use of very high doses of infliximab is clearly associated with a marked increase in the risk of infection.

If a child is running a fever or there are other reasons to suspect that there might be an infection, the dose of infliximab should not be given. Significant side effects of infliximab except for mild allergic reactions and infections are very rare, though all of the concerns related to altering the immune system with immunosuppressive medications should be considered. As with etanercept and adalimumab above, the ultimate duration of infliximab therapy is unclear.

Anakinra

Anakinra (sold as Kineret) is a novel biologic agent that works by blocking a messenger chemical called interleukin-1 (IL-1), preventing its attachment to the IL-1 receptor. The experience with anakinra in children is limited, but it has proven uniquely effective for many (though not all) children with systemic-onset juvenile arthritis. Also, there are children with psoriatic arthritis and with polyarticular juvenile arthritis who have responded to anakinra after failing to show improvement with other biologics.

Unlike infliximab, adalimumab, and etanercept, which are given less often, anakinra needs to be administered as a daily subcutaneous injection. It may be associated with abnormalities on routine blood tests and local pain at the injection site. It also has a slow onset of action. The combination of a slow onset of action and the need for daily injections limits its use in children who respond to other biologics. Anakinra has all of the side effects associated with other immunosuppressive drugs. Unfortunately, the combination of anakinra with etanercept resulted in an increased incidence of infections.

Although anakinra is effective, the ultimate place for this agent in the treatment of childhood arthritis is uncertain. In animal models, blocking IL-1 substantially reduced joint damage due to arthritis. For some children with systemic-onset disease anakinra has been miraculous, but for others it's ineffective. However, there is a group of genetic conditions, including neonatal onset multisystem inflammatory disease (NOMID) and Muckle-Wells syndrome, that respond dramatically and almost immediately to anakinra. Familial Mediterranean fever also responds well. Additional agents that block IL-1 but are given less frequently are under investigation and may ultimately replace anakinra.

Rituximab

Rituximab (marketed as Rituxan) was initially developed for the treatment of lymphomas. It is a monoclonal antibody directed against CD20, which is a surface marker present on activated B cells and perhaps some other lymphocytes, but not on mature plasma cells. When it was noted that some lymphoma patients who also had rheumatoid arthritis improved, studies of rituximab therapy for rheumatoid arthritis were begun.

It is now recognized the rituximab is effective in the treatment of rheumatoid arthritis, systemic lupus erythematosus, Wegener's granulomatosis, and dermatomyositis. It may prove effective in additional rheumatic diseases in the future. A number of studies are presently under way to determine the optimal regimen for the use of rituximab in each of these conditions. In adults with rheumatoid arthritis it is clear that rituximab may provide relief for severe cases that have not responded to TNF inhibitors. Rituximab has been very effective in children with rheumatoid-factor-positive arthritis when combined with cyclophosphamide or methotrexate. There is limited experience in other forms of juvenile arthritis, but it is likely to be beneficial. In adults with rheumatoid arthritis repeated treatment seems necessary, and this is likely to be true in children as well.

In adults and children with systemic lupus erythematosus the combination of rituximab and cyclophosphamide has often provided dramatic relief of symptoms and normalization of serologic parameters for prolonged periods. While the therapy is aggressive, a number of the children with SLE whom I treat have been able to wean themselves down to minimal doses of prednisone and remained ANA-negative for several years. The long-term safety and efficacy of this regimen are being studied.

One interesting aspect of rituximab therapy is that there is often an initial period of increased complaints lasting one or two months after the rituximab is given. However, this is followed by steady improvement in most children. The current regimen is to give two doses of rituximab (600 mg/m^2, up to 1,000 mg) two weeks apart (with or without cyclophosphamide) and repeat as necessary, but no more often than every four months. Therapy with rituximab depletes CD20-positive B cells and is associated with an increased risk of infection. Infusion reactions also may occur, and rituximab should be administered in an experienced infusion center. Most often corticosteroids and diphenhydramine are administered prior to the rituximab.

Abatacept

Abatacept (brand name Orencia) is a new agent that decreases the signaling between T cells and other cells in the immune system. Abatacept's mechanism of action is termed "co-stimulatory blockade." In the presence of infection, cells in the immune system interact to alert the immune system to the need for an inflammatory response. To minimize inappropriate messages, cells communicating with each other need to interact at several different levels: they need to be HLA-compatible, they need to be activated, and they need to interact with a co-stimulatory molecule (CD86). Abatacept blocks CD86 and thus decreases the inflammatory response.

There are studies of the use of abatacept in children with juvenile onset arthritis showing that it may be effective when the TNF inhibitors have not been. Whether it will prove to be most beneficial when used alone or in combination with other drugs is uncertain. There is also consideration of using abatacept in other childhood rheumatic diseases, but little information is available as I write this.

Newer Biologic Agents

There are several agents under development that may be available soon, but the uncertain nature of the final stages of clinical testing and governmental approval make this uncertain. One is a different agent to block IL-1 that has a different site of action and only needs to be given every two weeks. There are several drugs undergoing testing that block IL-6, a potent inflammatory mediator that is known to go up and down at the same time as the fever and rash come and go in children with severe systemic-onset arthritis. There are reports of excellent efficacy, but more information is needed regarding side effects.

OLDER IMMUNOSUPPRESSIVE AGENTS

Cyclosporine and Tacrolimus

Cyclosporine (marketed as Neoral or Sandimmune) and tacrolimus (marketed as Prograf) are closely related immunosuppressive drugs that are primarily used to prevent organ transplant rejection. Cyclosporine was discovered first and is used more widely, but tacrolimus may be more potent and have fewer side effects. However, there is only limited experience with the use of tacrolimus for arthritis at present, and so I restrict the rest of this discussion to cyclosporine.

Cyclosporine works primarily by blocking synthesis of IL-2 (a messenger molecule) and preventing the recruitment of additional inflammatory cells to a site of inflammation. It also affects IL-3, IL-4, and IFN-gamma, which are messenger molecules (cytokines) that promote inflammation. Since cyclosporine has an independent mechanism of action, in most cases it can be added to the other medications a child is taking.

Cyclosporine may be very beneficial in children with spondyloarthropathies, systemic-onset arthritis, arthritis associated with inflammatory bowel disease, dermatomyositis, and other vasculitic illnesses. It is also useful for the treatment of ocular inflammation (uveitis). However, a child's response to cyclosporine is unpredictable. Some children who have not responded to other medications have dramatically improved with the addition of cyclosporine. I have also used it in other children in seemingly identical situations without benefit.

Cyclosporine interferes with the immune system and has essentially the same risks as the other immunosuppressive drugs. The larger doses used to prevent organ transplant rejection are often associated with kidney damage (renal toxicity), but at the low dosages used for children with arthritis, this side effect is uncommon. However, children on cyclosporine should have all the normal monitoring tests with extra attention to make sure the urine and blood pressure are checked routinely. Changes in blood pressure or evidence of kidney irritation do occasionally occur at low doses, but with proper monitoring the drug can be discontinued as soon as they appear. In children who are carefully monitored, side effects are infrequent and generally resolve quickly with discontinuation of the drug.

Cyclosporine has several peculiarities. One is that it promotes hair growth not just on top of the head but elsewhere on the body. This may become unsightly, but if the cyclosporine is correcting the disease, it is acceptable.

Cyclosporine is also unusual in that it binds very strongly to glass. That means if you open the pills and put the medicine in a glass of water, the cyclosporine will bind to the glass and none will go into the child. Liquid cyclosporine is provided in a special container and must be administered directly to the child from that container. Another peculiarity is that children taking cyclosporine must avoid grapefruit juice, which contains a chemical that inactivates the drug.

Leflunomide

Leflunomide (marketed as Arava) is another of the immunosuppressive drugs that works by interfering with DNA synthesis. However, at the very low doses used by rheumatologists, it is suspected that leflunomide has other anti-inflammatory effects as well. In adult studies, leflunomide has proven effective for rheumatoid arthritis. It is a new drug, and at present the studies in children have not been published. I have had good results in teenagers with polyarticular arthritis and enthesitis-associated arthritis who have not been able to tolerate other agents. Most physicians feel that leflunomide is appropriately used only after methotrexate and perhaps one of the biologics has been tried. However, this is a matter of individual judgment.

Leflunomide can be added to NSAIDs and other medications. It does not act at the same point as methotrexate, so the two drugs can be combined, but either may cause liver and blood cell abnormalities and their combined use requires careful monitoring. As with other immunosuppressive drugs, leflunomide has a slow onset of action but appears to affect the course of the disease, not just relieve symptoms.

Leflunomide differs from most of the other immunosuppressive drugs in that it is ingested, processed by the liver, released from the liver into the intestine, and reabsorbed into the body from the intestine. Instead of being removed from the body, as are most drugs, the active part of leflunomide stays in the body for a long time. To take advantage of this, patients are given a big dose for the first few days, then a much smaller everyday dose. This is generally advantageous. However, if you need to get the drug out of the system (for example, because of a side effect) the child must be given cholestyramine, which binds to the leflunomide products in the intestine and prevents them from being reabsorbed. Once bound to cholestyramine, the active compounds are carried out of the body quickly.

Leflunomide requires careful monitoring of the child, just as with any other immunosuppressive drug. It may cause problems with the liver, the blood-forming cells, or elsewhere. It also may increase the risk of infection, as do the other immunosuppressive drugs. Diarrhea seems to be an occasional mild side effect. It seems less effective than methotrexate.

Mycophenolate Mofetil

Mycophenolate mofetil (marketed as Cellcept) is a newer immunosuppressive drug that inhibits DNA synthesis. It is primarily used for the treatment of organ transplant recipients but has been increasingly used for the treatment of children with SLE and other vasculitic diseases. It has also been used in children with uveitis and in adults with psoriatic arthritis. At present, the role of mycopheno-late mofetil in the treatment of children with arthritis has not yet been defined. It has been reported to be as effective as cyclophosphamide in high dosages, but most physicians have found the necessary dosage of mycophenolate mofetil to cause a significant incidence of stomach complaints, which force people to stop taking the medication. Too, practical clinical experience has not matched the success of the carefully selected patients in the published studies. More studies combining mycophenolate mofetil with other medications are under way.

Azathioprine

Azathioprine (Imuran), which works by inhibiting DNA synthesis, is one of the oldest of the immunosuppressive drugs. There is extensive experience using aza-thioprine in the treatment of children with arthritis and the vasculitic diseases. It has been useful in children with severe polyarticular-onset or systemic-onset JA. In the past, it was the primary immunosuppressive therapy, but with the widespread use of methotrexate, the biologics, leflunomide, and mycophenolate mofetil, there has been much less need for the use of azathioprine. It has all of the side effects of immunosuppressive drugs listed above. In addition, it is well known to sometimes cause liver irritation and problems with blood cell counts. It has also been associated with pancreatitis.

Cyclophosphamide

Cyclophosphamide (Cytoxan) is the most potent of the commonly used immu-nosuppressive agents. It is rarely used in the treatment of children with JA. Its use in the treatment of SLE is discussed in detail in Chapter 9. Cyclophosphamide can be given as daily pills or as intravenous injections. The intravenous injections are given on a variety of schedules, but the most common is monthly initially, then every three months until the course of therapy is completed. Except in special situations, daily pills should be avoided, as they have a much higher incidence of side effects than the intravenous injections.

Children receiving cyclophosphamide must be carefully monitored for evidence of bone marrow and bladder irritation. It is impractical to measure white blood cell counts and all other tests on a daily basis. If the medication is being given intravenously at intervals, all of the necessary tests can be done before each dose. Daily use of cyclophosphamide pills is associated with an increased risk of infection and a greatly increased risk of bladder damage. The damage to the bladder can lead to persistent bleeding and has been associated with the later development of bladder cancer.

Periodic intravenous injections of cyclophosphamide not only allow more careful monitoring but also allow the physician to make sure the child is well hydrated to prevent cyclophosphamide breakdown products from being allowed to sit in the bladder for a long period. In addition, most physicians administer MESNA intravenously after the cyclophosphamide. MESNA is a compound that binds to the cyclophosphamide breakdown products and neutralizes them. This reduces the risk of bladder irritation.

Intravenous cyclophosphamide has been used for the treatment of children with systemic-onset JA who failed all other therapies. Although there are a few reports in the literature describing success, it is not generally utilized because the treatment is difficult for the child and family and it is not universally successful. With the current availability of many new therapies, the role of cyclophosphamide in the treatment of children with arthritis is extremely limited. However, it remains a mainstay of therapy for children with vasculitic diseases, including SLE, dermatomyositis, and scleroderma. The future of cyclophosphamide in the therapy of rheumatic diseases may well lie in combining it with newer biologic agents, allowing a significant reduction in the total amount of cyclophosphamide given.

Chlorambucil

Chlorambucil (brand name Leukeran) is a very potent immunosuppressive agent that does not have the bladder-irritating properties of cyclophosphamide. It has been used for systemic-onset arthritis, vasculitic diseases, uveitis, and a variety of other life-threatening conditions. Chlorambucil does significantly impair the ability to deal with infections.

Chlorambucil is not widely used because it has been associated with the development of leukemia, sterility, and other complications far more often than the other immunosuppressive drugs discussed here. It should be considered only in the most difficult situations and used only by physicians with experience. Nonetheless, there are situations in which its use is appropriate.

CORTICOSTEROIDS

The discovery of corticosteroids was a major advance in the care of children and adults with rheumatic diseases. The beneficial effects of steroids result from their ability to block the effects of most inflammatory messengers (cytokines) and decrease the activity of the cells that promote inflammation. For children with severe diseases, the corticosteroids have vastly improved their quality of life. However, the excessive use of corticosteroids has many negative effects, and they should be used only when necessary. Excessive and unnecessary use of corticosteroids may cause great harm.

Steroids are simultaneously a blessing and a curse for children with JA. With a large enough dose of corticosteroids, virtually all of the manifestations of JA will rapidly disappear, but their continued usage causes an unacceptable level of side effects. These drugs may be absolutely necessary and life-saving under certain circumstances, but prolonged use in significant dosage is inevitably associated with complications.

With the ready availability of biologics, oral steroids should be necessary only in the treatment of systemic-onset JA, never pauciarticular-onset JA, and rarely polyarticular-onset JA. Corticosteroids are routinely used in the treatment of vasculitic diseases.

The adrenal gland in the body normally makes a certain amount of corticosteroids every day. If the adrenal gland fails, the result is a severe and life-threatening condition called Addison's disease. When your child takes extra corticosteroids every day, the body recognizes that there is no need for the adrenal gland to make more. If this continues for a long period, the adrenal gland may not be able to produce an adequate amount of corticosteroids. This is termed "adrenal suppression." There are two important consequences of adrenal suppression. First, if corticosteroids have been given long enough to shut down the adrenal gland (weeks, not days), they cannot be stopped abruptly. Instead, they must be withdrawn slowly to give the adrenal gland time to resume normal function.

Second, if your child is taking corticosteroids and becomes ill with nausea and vomiting, or if for any other reason your child cannot take the normal daily dose of corticosteroids, he or she needs to be given the dose by injection. This usually requires a visit to the doctor's office or the emergency room.

Even for children who have been able to discontinue corticosteroids, extra should be given if they need surgery or are under any form of significant physical stress, since their adrenal glands might not be able to produce the additional corticosteroids needed to deal with the stress. Make sure any doctor caring for your child knows that he or she is taking or has taken corticosteroids so that extra precautions can be taken if necessary.

Side Effects of Corticosteroids

The side effects of corticosteroids are numerous and very common. They include Cushing's syndrome, fluid retention, increased appetite and weight gain, truncal obesity (skinny arms and legs but increased fat on back and stomach), moon face (fat cheeks), stretch marks, acne, growth retardation, bone-weakening calcium loss, avascular necrosis, muscle weakness, poor blood sugar control (diabetes), cataracts, increased intraocular pressure, increased infections, oral and vaginal thrush, atherosclerosis, extra hair growth, and mood changes. In addition to these common side effects, corticosteroids also may cause high blood pressure, inflammation of the pancreas, and pseudotumor cerebrae (increased pressure in the brain, associated with severe headaches and visual problems).

Children with diseases such as SLE and dermatomyositis often must take corticosteroids (see Chapters 9 through 14), though the dosage should be minimized with use of immunosuppressive drugs. For children with systemic-onset JA with macrophage activation syndrome or other severe manifestations, corticosteroids are often mandatory. Most children with JA, however, should not be taking corticosteroids. The drugs should be reserved for those children with arthritis who cannot carry out their normal activities of daily living despite an adequate trial of other medications. In some cases the disease is evolving rapidly or has a significant head start and the child requires corticosteroids until another drug that can control the disease can take over and the steroids can be withdrawn.

A number of alternative regimens for the use of corticosteroids have been proposed. Many physicians have argued that given every other day, corticosteroids are less toxic. It is certainly true that 10 mg of prednisone every other day is less toxic than 10 mg every day. However, it is unclear that it is less toxic than 5 mg of prednisone every day, which may in fact be more effective. In some situations, physicians use high doses of corticosteroids given intravenously. This is thought to have fewer side effects than high daily oral doses of corticosteroids. On a one-time basis this is probably true. However, this has not proven to be true when the high intravenous doses are given routinely.

Intra-articular Corticosteroids

Triamcinolone (Aristospan), betamethasone (Celestone), and methylprednisone (Depo-Medral) are corticosteroid preparations often used for intra-articular injections, where the drug is injected directly into the inflamed joint. MRIs have shown that these injections have a very positive effect on reducing the inflammation and promoting healing of the cartilage. However, it is important that children not resume activities that may be harmful to their joints simply because the injections have made them feel better.

Intra-articular corticosteroid injections should be considered for a child with a single swollen joint who is not responding well to NSAIDs. Studies even suggest that the liberal use of intra-articular injections has reduced the frequency of leg-length discrepancy in children with true pauciarticular-onset arthritis. Since the therapy is generally safe and effective, it should probably be done sooner than later.

A number of physicians believe it is appropriate to anesthetize a child with three or four swollen joints and then inject each of the joints. It is true the children will feel much better for a period of days after several joints are injected because the corticosteroids slowly leak out of the joints and have a systemic effect, just as if they were taken by mouth (this effect is minimal if only a single joint is injected). It is my belief that if there are more than two swollen joints, it means that the disease is not under adequate control. These children should be given better systemic medication instead of multiple joint injections.

I normally do not anesthetize children for joint injections, as anesthesia carries its own set of medications and risks. However, it can be done at the family's request. Since I rarely do more than one joint, I find joint injections to be a quick and easy procedure. The skin around the joint to be injected is cleaned. Numbing medicine can be injected around the area of the joint (this burns a little and I give children the choice of skipping it). Then the physician simply slips the needle into the joint and injects the corticosteroids. Although children up to age twelve or so will need to be helped to hold still when it hurts, most children tolerate this very well with positive reassurance from parents and the doctor. I always tell children it will hurt for a minute and challenge them to see if they can say "Ouch" louder than I can. In the distraction of listening to me say "Ouch," many of them forget to.

It is very difficult to predict for how long an intra-articular joint injection will provide relief. Sometimes there is only a single involved knee, and after it is injected the child never has trouble again. Other times the knee is injected and there is no apparent improvement. Most often joint injections provide two or three months of relief and allow other medications to take effect and control the disease. A frequent need for joint injections suggests that the child's disease is not being adequately controlled by the systemic medications.

There are very few risks associated with intra-articular joint injections. The greatest risk is that associated with anesthesia if children are anesthetized. Other risks associated with intra-articular joint injections include the risk of an infection as the result of being injected, an unusual "crystal reaction" to the injected medication, and damage to the skin around the injection site. If corticosteroids leak into the skin and adjacent tissues during the injection, they cause loss of fat under the skin, causing something that looks like a dimple.

Whenever a joint is injected, it is important for the physician to use a short-acting agent such as betamethasone if the area being injected is close to the surface (a tendon, a finger, or a wrist joint), to minimize the risk of skin damage. Long-lasting agents such as triamcinolone should be reserved for large joints such as knees and hips.

There has been a lot of discussion about how much to limit activities after injecting a large joint. The goal is to suppress the inflammation for as long as possible. To accomplish this, the injected corticosteroids should remain in the joint for as long as possible. Ideally, the child is not active for the first twenty-four hours after the injection. Some physicians even go so far as to place a temporary cast on the leg if the knee is injected, removing it the next day. Most of us settle for instructing the family to limit unnecessary activities for twenty-four hours.

It is also necessary to remember that the corticosteroids to be injected are typically mixed with lidocaine, an anesthetic. Be sure to tell the physician if your child is allergic to lidocaine. The mixture of corticosteroid and lidocaine has the advantage of immediately making the joint numb, reducing pain. However, since the joint will be numb for several hours after the injection, a child could injure the injected joint and not know it.

MISCELLANEOUS AGENTS

Thalidomide

Thalidomide (Thalomid) is a medication that was initially used as a sedative. It was withdrawn from the market in the early 1960s, just a few years after its release, because it causes significant birth defects if taken by pregnant women. It was subsequently discovered to have very potent anti-inflammatory effects. Although parents and physicians initially are concerned on learning that thalidomide is known to cause birth defects, none of the immunosuppressive drugs is safe to give to pregnant women. Fortunately, in pediatric rheumatology, pregnancy is rarely an immediate concern. There is no evidence that thalidomide has any lingering effects more than a month after it is discontinued. Thalidomide is very effective for some children with systemic-onset, psoriatic, and polyarticular-onset arthritis who have not responded to other medications.

Thalidomide may cause abnormalities in the routine blood tests, including decreased white blood cell count and elevated liver enzymes, and so monitoring is required. Thalidomide is associated with nerve irritation that can produce pain and tingling. This should be monitored for. Continued treatment with thalidomide could result in permanent nerve damage. However, in the dosage recommended for children with arthritis this has not been a significant problem. Thalidomide also causes an increase in the risk of blood clotting. This has been a minor problem in adults receiving thalidomide for multiple myeloma, and physicians treating children with systemic-onset arthritis should be aware of the possibility.

The use of thalidomide currently requires extensive monitoring to ensure that the patient is not at risk for becoming pregnant. Although it seems improbable for small children, one can never be too careful. At the present time in the United States, only physicians who have registered with the company that provides the drug can prescribe thalidomide.

This drug may become more important in the future because it downregulates the genes that are responsible for synthesis of many inflammatory molecules (that is, the drug signals the genes to make fewer of them).

Intravenous Gamma Globulin

Intravenous gamma globulin (IV IgG) received a lot of attention in the early 1990s. It is still used for many diseases by some physicians, but the cost is extremely high and its use has largely been supplanted by the biologics. Some physicians still believe this is an excellent medication for dermatomyositis. It is very effective for children with Kawasaki disease (see Chapter 15). The difference is that Kawasaki disease is an acute illness. Once you have treated a child for Kawasaki disease with IV IgG, in most cases the illness is cured.

The effect of IV IgG seems to decrease with each successive dose. Children with a chronic disease treated with IV IgG often seemed much improved initially, but they would require more and more IV IgG over time (and usually more frequent treatment) with less and less effect. As a result, the benefits of IV IgG for chronic conditions such as arthritis and dermatomyositis are less clear. It is a useful therapy for children with immune deficiency diseases who do not make enough of their own IgG, because in those cases it is simply a replacement therapy.

Significant negative side effects may occur with the use of IV IgG. This therapy must be given as periodic intravenous infusions and may be associated with allergic reactions. In general, this therapy should be restricted to specific situations such as Kawasaki disease and some hematologic disorders.

"Gold Shots"

Gold sodium thioglucose and gold sodium thiomalate (brand names Myochrysine and Solganol, also known as "gold shots") were the standard of therapy for difficult arthritis in adults and children when I began my career. For many children, they were dramatically effective, bringing a slow but steady resolution of the arthritis. The major difficulty with gold shots is that they require painful intramuscular injections. The injections are given weekly until the arthritis is well under control and then slowly spaced out over longer intervals.

Since gold shots can have significant impact on the blood-forming cells, most physicians do routine blood work before every dose. Frequent testing and doctor visits are a major inconvenience. Side effects beyond the inconvenience of frequent physician visits were most often limited to minor changes in the blood tests. Severe side effects do occur, but they are infrequent.

Over the past twenty years, most physicians have replaced the use of gold shots with methotrexate and now the new biologics. Methotrexate is usually given in oral form and is far more convenient. It is unclear where gold shots belong in the current approach to therapy. There are many children whose arthritis disappeared when they were treated with gold shots. However, some children ultimately relapsed after the gold shots were discontinued. The biologics, such as etanercept, clearly provide a quicker and greater level of relief with less apparent toxicity. I almost never use gold shots now, but there may still be a place for them.

Auranofin

Auranofin (Ridaura) is an oral version of gold salts given as daily pills. It was developed in an effort to overcome the inconvenience associated with weekly gold shots. Unfortunately, auranofin does not seem to be as effective as gold shots, though it has just as many side effects. It is rarely if ever used in childhood.

D-Penicillamine

D-penicillamine clearly affects the course of JA, morphea, and scleroderma, but it has a very slow onset of action and a high frequency of toxic reactions (routine blood test abnormalities, skin rashes, kidney irritation, and neurologic abnormalities). Because of these drawbacks, D-penicillamine was rapidly replaced by methotrexate for the treatment of children with arthritis. D-penicillamine may still have a role for children who have not responded to other medications, but it is rare to see it used for arthritis in childhood.

D-penicillamine has long been the standard recommended therapy for children with morphea and scleroderma (progressive systemic sclerosis). Although some physicians report good effects, most physicians with extensive experience find D-penicillamine to have a high frequency of toxicity and only minimal efficacy. The right therapy for scleroderma remains controversial, but I prefer methotrexate. For most children with scleroderma or morphea, methotrexate has greater efficacy and less toxicity than D-penicillamine. Nevertheless, there are well-respected physicians who continue to use D-penicillamine for scleroderma.

OTHER MODALITIES: PLASMAPHARESIS

Plasmapharesis (also called apharesis) is a technique by which the patient's blood is removed from the body so the plasma (the clear fluid left after the blood's cells are removed) can be removed and replaced, while the blood cells are returned to the patient. If there is a toxic element in the plasma, plasmapharesis will remove it.

At one point, plasmapharesis was considered a possible therapy for a wide variety of diseases. However, it was found to lack lasting beneficial effects. Today, plasmapharesis is not routinely used for the therapy of children with any rheumatic disease. However, it is occasionally beneficial for crisis management in children with systemic lupus erythematosus or antiphospholipid antibody syndrome. Controlled studies do not convincingly show any sustained benefit from plasmapharesis after the acute crisis. Over time, the toxic effects mount, while the therapeutic efficacy decreases.

IMMUNIZATIONS

Routine Vaccinations

The most important thing to understand about immunizations is that they have saved millions of lives. Routine vaccination against smallpox eliminated a terrible and often fatal disease from the world. Although it may take a full generation, routine immunization against hepatitis B will also save hundreds of thousands of lives. You will find it nearly impossible to locate a young American doctor with experience treating polio, measles, mumps, rubella, or their complications because routine vaccination has made these diseases very rare. At present, every American child is routinely vaccinated against polio, tetanus, measles, mumps, rubella, pertussis (whooping cough), and hepatitis B.

To meet the current recommendations of the American Academy of Pediatrics, children receive at least fifteen vaccinations during the first three years of life. Pauciarticular-onset juvenile arthritis frequently starts in young children in this age group, so chances are that children develop the disease within a few months of a vaccination. Since certain injections can cause a fever and pain, it is natural for parents of a child with arthritis to suspect that the injection may have played a role.

A proper study would require evaluating the frequency of juvenile arthritis in a large group of children who did not get properly vaccinated. However, it would be unethical to do this. What I can tell you is that I have been practicing for more than twenty-five years, some of that in areas where routine vaccinations were not always done because people did not come to the doctor. There does not appear to be any increase in the incidence of juvenile arthritis among properly vaccinated children. We know there are small risks associated with routine vaccination, but the risks of the diseases we are being protected against are far more severe.

However, while I believe it is important that all normal children receive vaccinations, the situation for children who already have arthritis is more complicated. Here there is a diversity of opinion among doctors. In addition, the answer depends on what medications your child is taking. What I am stating here are only my own views.

Most often your child will have received polio, tetanus, measles, mumps, and rubella immunizations before developing arthritis. Although several doses of vaccine are recommended, children get some protection from even a single dose. A child who has never been vaccinated against these diseases is a special case that will require careful consideration between the parents and physician.

If a child has received the three routine vaccinations scheduled up to six months of age and the first MMR (measles, mumps, rubella) vaccination, then the child should not receive any further vaccines while the arthritis is active. For children who are off medications or taking only a routine NSAID and if the arthritis has been fully controlled for six months, then one can carefully consider giving vaccinations.

Rubella is the only vaccine that routinely causes transient arthritis as a side effect. I would check to see whether a child has a reasonable titer of immunity (this is a routine blood test) and not revaccinate with rubella if the child is immune. I would avoid live vaccines (e.g., the chickenpox vaccine [herpes zoster] and the smallpox vaccine) in any child who has active disease or is receiving immunosuppressive drugs. These recommendations are detailed in the box.

A major issue that is often overlooked by physicians and families is the possible spread of a disease from live virus vaccines among people with close contact. If your child is receiving medications that impede the ability to fight infection (including but not limited to corticosteroids, methotrexate, and biologics), not only should the child not receive live vaccines, but neither should the child's brothers and sisters. The altered virus contained in these vaccines can spread from one child to another and cause severe problems in an immunologically compromised child. You must also be careful about letting your child come in close contact with other children who have been recently vaccinated.

Recommendations for Vaccinations in Children with Rheumatic Disease

Child with arthritis who are off all medications and have been well for six months or more

All vaccines recommended may be given, but avoid rubella if the child has a positive titer, indicating immunity to rubella.

Child with arthritis who is on NSAIDs but has been well for six months

Most routine vaccinations are okay, but avoid rubella if the child has a positive titer. Do not give any live-virus vaccines (e.g., chicken pox [herpes zoster] and smallpox), as there is risk of disease and Reye's syndrome.

Child with arthritis who is on immunosuppressive medications (corticosteroids, etanercept, infliximab, anakinra, adalimumab) or cytotoxics (methotrexate, mycophenolate mofetil, cyclophosphamide, azathioprine)

Do not give the child any vaccinations. However, there are data suggesting that pneumococcal vaccine should be given if it hasn't already been. No live-virus vaccinations should be given to siblings or household contacts.

Child with active arthritis within the past six months (no matter what the medications)

No vaccinations should be given to the child (note that not all doctors agree on this). This has to be reviewed on a case-by-case basis when issues such as college dormitory life, travel, or risk of epidemic exposure arise.

Other Vaccines

Flu shots. The consensus opinion is that the benefits outweigh the risks. I let parents make their own decision.

Pneumococcal vaccine. It is now recommended by the American Academy of Pediatrics that young children receive the pneumococcal vaccine (Pneumovax) vaccination early in life. It prevents many types of serious pneumonia and other infections caused by the same family of bacteria. Most older children have not gotten it. It should be given to children if you think you are going to put them on immunosuppressive medications, but it must be given before you start the immunosuppressive medication for it to be most effective. There is evidence that it still has some benefit even if the children are on immunosuppressive medicine. This is safe because it is not a live vaccine.

Meningococcal vaccine. The meningococcal vaccine, which protects against meningitis, is frequently recommended for college freshman and increasingly for even younger children.

Human papillomavirus (HPV). The newly introduced HPV vaccine (Gardasil) is being recommended for girls to reduce the risk of cervical cancer. There is some concern that it may stimulate the immune system enough to cause increased complaints in children with rheumatic disease, but preventing cervical cancer is an important goal that rheumatologists feel justifies any increased arthritis-related problems.

Bird flu. The reports in the media have become less frequent, but as I write this bird flu is still a significant problem for birds, though only rarely for people. Should there be a new pandemic because bird flu does become an easily contagious human disease, the benefits of immunization with a satisfactory killed-virus vaccine will outweigh the risks of increased arthritis.

Smallpox (vaccinia). Smallpox was and still is a terrible condition that is often fatal. Worldwide vaccination programs have led to the elimination of this disease except as a biowarfare threat. This is a live-virus vaccine and has a significant risk of causing trouble to anyone who is immunosuppressed. It is also a member of the herpes family of viruses, which has been linked to Reye's syndrome.

Should the disease ever again become a real threat, it will be necessary to immunize as many people as possible. For children on NSAIDs only, the risk would be acceptable under those circumstances. For children on immunosuppressive drugs, it would be necessary to stop those drugs at least fourteen days before vaccination and maintain the child off the drugs for a month after the vaccination. (If the Centers for Disease Control make official recommendations for this situation, we should follow them; so far they have not.) The risks of doing this will have to be considered for each child's situation.

21

Alternative Medicine

Vitamins, Supplements, and Other Treatments

You cannot treat illness without the risk of side effects. Whether you take the prescribed medications, buy over-the-counter medications, ignore the problem and hope it will go away, buy a supplement in a health food store, or try a "cure" from some other source, there are risks associated with every choice. The only difference is whether or not those risks are clearly explained to you. The physician is required to tell you about potential side effects for medications, and warnings are printed on the labels of over-the-counter medications for you to read, but for any other substance you're on your own.

There are many things to remember when you consider using supplements or alternative medicines. First and foremost is that none of these is subject to any regulation regarding the truth of their claims, the purity of the product, or even that what it says on the label is what is in the product. Many supplements have been found to contain little if any of the ingredients highlighted on the label, and some have been found to be contaminated with heavy metals and other known harmful substances.

READ THE LABEL CAREFULLY AND DON'T BELIEVE EVERYTHING YOU HEAR

It is with dismay that I see parents bring in all sorts of things found in health food stores, noted on the Internet, advertised on television, or seen in the newspaper. Sometimes they even bring in a vitamin or supplement that another doctor was selling in his or her office (though this was declared unethical by several medical societies and may soon be illegal). The parents want me to say that it's all right to give it to their child. Most would not be fooled for a moment if the item promised stock market riches or a new way to keep your car from needing gasoline, but when it comes to their child's health, they want very much to believe that miracle cures exist. The fact is that there are lots of unscrupulous individuals out there who will sell you anything to get your money.

Health aids are a billion-dollar-a-year business. Most are harmless except for the expense, and some may have a positive placebo effect (see below). However, some are potentially harmful, especially for people who really do have a medical problem. Moreover, their use may delay proper diagnosis and treatment. There are no rules restricting what salespeople can say in stores or what can be claimed on the Internet. The small print on labels always says, "These statements have not been evaluated by the Food and Drug Administration. This product is not intended to diagnose, treat, cure, or prevent any disease." By contrast, FDA-approved drugs are made in factories that are carefully inspected. The medications are checked to be sure that they are really what they say they are and to be sure they contain no contaminants that could be harmful. They are prescribed by licensed physicians who have been trained in their use and who do not have a financial incentive for you to take the drug.

Many people assume that physicians are automatically against anything they did not prescribe. Literature on alternative medicine may even contain a statement such as "Doctors are not going to give you this because it will cure you. Then you will not have to go back and they will not make any money." Nothing could be further from the truth. If peanut butter from the supermarket cured arthritis, I'd be thrilled to send my patients straight to the checkout counter. In the sections that follow, I discuss vitamin and mineral supplementation, alternative diets, dietary supplements, and herbal cures. Some I favor; others I oppose.

When you meet someone who is sure that a special diet or supplement made his or her arthritis better, remember the person may or may not have the same disease your child has. Second, large-scale studies of adults with arthritis have clearly documented a substantial placebo effect. In studies of new medications, patients are divided into two groups. One group gets the new medication; the other gets an identical-appearing sugar pill. In virtually every such study, one-third of the patients receiving the sugar pill report dramatic improvement. They are not lying. They feel better. Whether this was due to spontaneous improvement, psychological effects, or other factors varied from patient to patient. But the sugar pills did not make them better.

Before you consider any alternative therapy for your child, ask yourself the following questions:

- Would you accept a prescription for the same thing from your doctor?
- Have you ever heard of the manufacturer?
- Is any proof supplied for the claims made? Can that proof be independently verified?
- Where was it made? Is the facility certified by any reputable organization?
- Who is recommending this and what is that person's training?
- Will the person recommending it make a profit if you buy this?
- If you are going to make your child take this, would you take it yourself?
- What do you know about possible side effects or possible interference with the medicines your child is supposed to be taking?
- Have you discussed this with your child's doctor?

If you're afraid to discuss with the doctor any alternative treatments you want to give your child, either do not give the treatment or find a doctor you are not afraid to talk to. I discuss these things with my patients all the time. If it's essentially harmless, I'll tell them so. I stop families from doing things or giving children things only if I believe they are unsafe.

VITAMINS

Every child with chronic disease should be on a daily vitamin that contains the appropriate amounts of vitamins A, B (all types), C, D, E, and K, folic acid, iron, and calcium. Children with iron deficiency, whether from inadequate intake, from chronic blood loss, or because their bodies don't utilize iron well, may need additional iron supplementation. However, iron-containing medications may cause upset stomach, and overdosage of iron can be harmful and possibly even fatal, so keep the pills in a safe place and give extra iron (more than a regular multivitamin contains) only on a doctor's advice.

Calcium is necessary, but in excess it causes upset stomach and constipation. In severe excess, calcium can also contribute to kidney stones (especially if combined with a lot of vitamin C).

Most vitamins have a tremendous safety range. However, vitamins A and D are stored in the body and may reach toxic levels. Too much vitamin A or D can cause severe illness and even death.

When you buy your vitamins I strongly recommend you stick with an established brand from a major national manufacturer. Not all vitamin pills are the same. Some pills will claim a large amount of an ingredient, but it may not be in a form your body can use. In addition, you have no way of knowing what the filler in the vitamin is or what it may be contaminated with.

SUPPLEMENTS

If you decide to give your child supplements, I advise the same caution as I do for vitamins: choose an established brand from a major national manufacturer.

Glucosamine

One supplement that has been shown to be of benefit for people with osteoarthritis, which is due to the breakdown of cartilage with age, is glucosamine. Glucosamine is a raw ingredient used by the body in manufacturing cartilage. However, osteoarthritis is not the cause of the problems in children with arthritis. Still, the side effects of glucosamine are usually mild. In contrast, chondroitin sulfate, which is often marketed with glucosamine, has failed to show benefit in studies and has been shown to cause an increased frequency of stomach upset.

Essential Fatty Acids (Omega-3, Omega-6)

Omega-3 fatty acids are oils found in large amounts in cold-water fish. These fatty acids alter the synthesis of inflammatory mediators in the body. However, to achieve that effect it's necessary to take ten or more capsules every day.

Research has shown that many adults with rheumatoid arthritis who take omega-3s show significant improvement after six to eight weeks of taking the supplement. However, by twelve weeks the body readjusts itself and begins to make increased amounts of the inflammatory mediators again, so there seem to be no long-term benefits. The major side effects of omega-3 fatty acids are increased bruising and prolonged bleeding. It's also very expensive if you take the amount necessary to show a short-term effect.

Flaxseed oil is another source of essential fatty acids that is frequently recommended for the treatment of arthritis. There is no long list of negative side effects, but there is no convincing evidence it helps, either.

Other sources have suggested that evening primrose oil, black currant oil, and borage oil, which contain omega-6 fatty acids, may be beneficial. However, all of these products have failed to demonstrate a positive effect when compared with placebo, and they may cause side effects.

DIET

Many different sources recommend that people with arthritis should avoid all sorts of foods: vegetables in the nightshade family (white potatoes, tomatoes, eggplant, peppers), red meat, any meat, gluten, mushrooms, and many more. Putting a child on a special diet may seem to parents like a way of taking control over an illness that can make them feel powerless in the face of their child's suffering.

I never argue with a family that tells me they have adopted a special diet and the child feels better (as long as it is a healthy diet). However, large-scale testing has not shown any of these diets to be particularly beneficial for children with arthritis. The only exception is children with celiac disease. These children may develop arthritis as one manifestation of their disease and will do better on a low-gluten diet. If you are unsure, double-check that your child has been checked for this; the initial screening is a simple blood test. Most will not have celiac disease, but we need to find the few who do.

From time to time I see children who have been placed on strict elimination diets because the family believes the arthritis is due to a food allergy. Although families sometimes convince themselves of short-term benefits, I've never seen a child get better over the long term because of these diets. They put your child through useless deprivation and can negatively affect the child's physical growth and self-image.

ALTERNATIVE MEDICAL SYSTEMS

We've all probably heard stories of people who got better after they prayed to a certain saint, went to Lourdes, had acupuncture done, or took up Zen. Thirty years of caring for children with rheumatic disease have made it clear to me that I cannot always explain why their symptoms get better or worse on a given day. The diseases do wax and wane over time. Sometimes people are going to get lucky and get better right after doing something unlikely to really help. Arguing with them that it was a coincidence probably will have no effect—they know they got better, and they will try to convince you to do the same thing. Be very careful. If anything worked consistently, we'd all be recommending it. But I have seen lots of families who took their children to Lourdes, the Dead Sea, or the acupuncturist with no effect. If something worked more often than random chance, I'd be telling you about it. In this era of global travel and communication, there is no hidden cure being used in some remote part of the world that we do not know about. I frequently teach in Asia and Africa, and the question there is always whether I can help them get more American medicines. No one has ever come up to me and said, "Here, take this stuff home, it will cure everyone."

22

Understanding Laboratory and Diagnostic Tests

In this chapter I discuss the most common laboratory and diagnostic tests. There are a number of less commonly used diagnostic tests that are specific to different diseases; rather than discuss each of them here, I have included them in the sections related to those diseases where they are relevant. If you have concerns about a test not discussed here, ask your physician for more information.

X-RAYS

If a bone is painful, it is appropriate to begin the evaluation (after a complete history is taken and a thorough physical examination is done) with an X-ray to eliminate the possibility of fracture or structural abnormality. X-rays are also useful to determine whether bones are out of alignment or abnormally curved. An X-ray may be the only study necessary to establish the diagnosis of a broken bone, slipped capital femoral epiphysis, scoliosis, or any of a number of other orthopedic conditions. However, for children with juvenile arthritis, lupus, or many other rheumatic conditions, the X-ray may be useful only to exclude orthopedic problems or if there is any history of trauma before the onset of pain. The bones are not fully calcified in young children, and the use of X-rays to evaluate arthritis in them is of little value except in the most severe cases.

Once the initial X-rays have been done, follow up X-rays are necessary only if a fracture is suspected, if there is a structural abnormality that must be monitored, if there is a sudden change, or if the problem is not resolving in the expected manner.

While exposure to unnecessary X-rays should be avoided, today's X-rays expose a child to far less radiation than was the case years ago, and the risk to the child is minimal. The potential risk of undetected disease is far greater.

CAT SCANS

In a CAT (computed axial tomography) scan, X-rays that pass through the body are recorded by a computer that creates a three-dimensional picture.

These pictures may reveal far greater detail than regular X-rays and provide a lot of additional information.

MRI

In magnetic resonance imaging (MRI), a machine locates specific types of molecules in the body, most often water molecules. The machines are calibrated so that they can detect differences in the concentration of water molecules in different tissues; a computer program uses these data to construct a picture of the tissues. MRI is excellent for imaging soft tissues of the body. Bone marrow contains water and shows up well, as does the cartilage covering the ends of the bones; the bones themselves contain little water and do not show up well. An MRI does not involve X-rays.

BONE SCANS, GALLIUM SCANS, PET SCANS

Bone scans are based on the uptake of the radioactive isotope technetium-99 (Tc-99) by active bone cells. Normal bone cells are not very active, but if there is an injury, arthritis, infection, or tumor, the bone cells become active in trying to repair the damage, and so they take up more calcium and related substances. When Tc-99 is injected, active bone cells take it up. Because it is radioactive, a picture of where it went in the body can be made using a gamma counter. Bone scans can find problem areas that are too small to be obvious on regular X-rays or CAT scans. It can also find areas where the bone cells have been irritated but obvious changes have not taken place. As a result, this test is very good for finding things such as osteomyelitis (bone infections) and osteoid osteomas (small, benign bone tumors) before they are evident on X-ray. Although the actual lesion may not be large, the irritated bone will show up quite brightly. One advantage of a bone scan is that it allows the physician to evaluate the entire body for areas of bone irritation with a single test.

Where inflammation of soft tissue is suspected, a similar scan can be done with radioactive gallium-67 (Ga-67). Inflamed tissue in the liver, spleen, lung, muscle, and other tissues take up the radioactive gallium to a greater degree than normal tissues, helping physicians to locate infections, tumors, and other problems. As with the bone scan, this has the advantage of allowing the evaluation of the entire body with a single test.

Although bone scans and gallium scans are done using the same machinery, they cannot be done simultaneously. Bone scans are completed the same day as the radioactive isotope, and the Tc-99 is rapidly removed from the body. The gallium scan procedure is done over a period of three days because the Ga-67 takes longer to reach the tissues and also longer to leave the body. As a result, if both tests are necessary, it is important to do the bone scan first. The gallium scan can then be started the next day. It is necessary to wait more than a week after a gallium scan has been done (for the Ga-67 to clear the system) before a bone scan can be done.

Nuclear medicine specialists have begun to recommend PET (positron emission tomography) scans, which detect areas of increased cellular activity due to increased sugar uptake. This is faster than gallium scanning and may ultimately replace it.

As with X-rays, it would be foolish to expose anyone unnecessarily to radioactive isotopes. However, dosages of the isotopes are kept to the absolute minimum necessary, and the risk to children who have these tests is generally negligible. The risk of undetected disease is far greater than the risk of damage from the test.

DIAGNOSTIC ULTRASOUND (SONOGRAPHY)

Ultrasound is a relatively new technology that may allow us to study muscles, bones, and joints at far less cost and without the risks associated with radiation. At the present time, the use of ultrasound to evaluate joint swelling and tendon inflammation is rapidly advancing. These tests may be available to your doctor and may be quite helpful in evaluating problems in the muscles and joints. Ultrasound can also be used to guide the doctors when they need to inject joints they cannot see, such as the hips.

SYNOVIAL FLUID ASPIRATION

Synovial fluid aspiration, or the removal of fluid from an inflamed joint, is often done in the physician's office. However, sometimes it is done in the radiology department because physicians want to use X-ray guidance or ultrasound to make sure the needle is in the right place. Synovial fluid aspiration is normally done for the purpose of analyzing the fluid to look for evidence of infection, bleeding, or tumors. In children, the test is done most often to exclude the possibility of infection. Even children who are known to have arthritis can develop an infection in the joint.

The fluid removed is subjected to a number of tests, including measurements of protein and sugar. For the cell count, less than 5,000 cells is considered normal. A cell count of 5,000 to 50,000 is consistent with arthritis but can also be seen with Lyme disease and irritation of the joint. A count of 50,000 to 100,000 may indicate arthritis, Lyme disease, or an infection. More than 100,000 cells indicates probable infection.

A gram stain to look for bacteria is always done no matter what the cell count is, and some of the fluid should be sent for culture by the bacteriology laboratory. If tuberculosis is a possibility, special stains should be done on the fluid (it won't show up on the gram stain) and special culture techniques must be used.

In adults, doctors look for crystals in synovial fluid, which can help detect gout and pseudo-gout. However, neither of these diseases occurs in children under normal circumstances.

If the synovial fluid is bloody, it may indicate that a vessel was nicked during the procedure. However, if this is the case, the blood will be fresh (tests can distinguish fresh blood from old blood). There is an uncommon disease called pigmented villonodular synovitis that causes bleeding into the joint. Usually, this is suspected when there is evidence of old blood in the joint. Old blood in the synovial fluid may also come from an injury.

One important source of error in evaluating synovial fluid may occur when the end of the bone near the joint is infected. In this situation the child may be complaining of knee pain, but the synovial fluid does not reveal evidence of an infection in the joint. Careful physical examination can reveal the bone infection. Infection will not show up on an X-ray until it is well established; however, a bone scan or MRI will reveal the infection even at the earliest stages.

When a child with a swollen joint is scheduled for synovial fluid aspiration, parents often wonder why the physicians do not simply take all the fluid out while they have a needle in the joint. Unfortunately, the fluid will rapidly reappear. Medications are needed to stop the production of the fluid.

PULMONARY FUNCTION TESTING

Pulmonary function testing (PFT) is a special set of tests to measure the child's ability to breathe. The first part of the test measures the ability of the lungs to move air in and out. This part of the test may be repeated after a medication called a bronchodilator is given, which reverses changes due to constriction of the airways by asthma or a similar illness. If the tests improve after the child uses a bronchodilator, part of the problem may be asthma or a similar disease.

Obstructive lung disease occurs when something is getting in the way of the air flow. This is rare in children with rheumatic disease. Restrictive lung disease describes when the lungs themselves are not moving well. This can be due to weakness, but more often it means the lungs themselves are stiff. Most often, this happens when the lungs are involved by scleroderma, but it can happen with other rheumatic diseases.

The second part of the PFT measures the ability of the lungs to move oxygen from the air inhaled into the lungs to the blood passing through the lungs. If the child is not getting enough oxygen, he or she will feel out of breath all the time.

LABORATORY TESTS

Lab test results must be viewed as part of the total picture of the patient, along with a good history and physical examination. Many rheumatic diseases are associated with abnormal laboratory tests, but there are diseases in which all the tests are normal. Conversely, many children are found to have mild laboratory abnormalities but do not have rheumatic disease. It is also important to remember that laboratory tests are not always accurate. Always recheck a result that does not make sense, or a key result that would change the course of treatment if it does not fit the clinical picture.

CBC and MCV

A complete blood count (CBC) is one of the most routine blood tests, yet it provides a lot of useful information.

Hemoglobin and hematocrit. These measure the amount of red blood cells in the blood (albeit in different units). If the child has a low hemoglobin or hematocrit, he or she is anemic. The anemia may be from many different causes but should prompt further investigation.

RBC, RDW, MCV, MCH, and MCHC. These parts of the CBC help differentiate causes of anemia. In general, only the mean corpuscular volume (MCV), which describes the size of the red blood cells, is important in bone and joint conditions. When the MCV is very low (the red blood cells are too small), usually it is because there is not enough hemoglobin in the cells. This is most often the result of iron deficiency, which can be confirmed with two additional tests, a measure of iron in the blood (Fe) and total iron bind capacity (TIBC). It can also be caused by genetic diseases in which hemoglobin is not properly made, such as thalassemia. In rheumatic diseases, the MCV is often low.

A high MCV may indicate an increased number of young red blood cells called reticulocytes, which can be caused by iron deficiency, deficiency of the vitamin folate (which can be caused by the drugs sulfasalazine and methotrexate, commonly used by rheumatologists), or hemolytic anemia (in which the body rapidly destroys red blood cells because of a metabolic or autoimmune problem and the bone marrow attempts to compensate by releasing large numbers of reticulocytes, which are larger than mature red blood cells). Hemolytic anemia may be an isolated problem, but it may also be caused by a number of rheumatic conditions, including systemic lupus erythematosus. Hemolytic anemia can also be caused by medications, and occurs with increased frequency in children who lack an enzyme found in normal red blood cells called G6PD. G6PD deficiency, which can be detected with a separate test, is more common in children of African, Asian, Middle Eastern, or Mediterranean heritage. Hydroxychloroquine is a commonly used drug in pediatric rheumatology that may cause problems for children who are G6PD-deficient.

The automated machine that performs the CBC typically produces an average MCV reading. Thus, young cells that are large and old cells that are small may average out to a normal number despite low hemoglobin. However, this situation can be detected easily by ordering a reticulocyte count to identify the young cells. (Some newer machines used to do CBCs will detect this situation automatically.)

WBC. White blood cells are a critical component of the body's defense against infection. If the count goes too high, it suggests that that child is under physiologic stress. Infection is one of the possible causes of this type of stress. However, certain medications will make the count go up as well. Very high WBC counts can occur in diseases such as juvenile arthritis (especially systemic-onset juvenile arthritis), severe infections, and leukemia (cancer of the white blood cells).

A low white blood cell count (WBC) is called leukopenia. If the white count goes too low, the child is vulnerable to infections. Low WBC counts can be the result of leukemia (if the cancerous white blood cells are not being released into the circulation) or systemic lupus erythematosus. More often a low WBC count is the result of medications or certain viral infections. Many of the medications used in treating children with rheumatic diseases cause low WBC counts. A rare cause of very low WBC counts is a condition called aplastic anemia, in which the bone marrow elements that make the white blood cells (and others) fail. Whenever a child's count is too low, careful attention should be given to all of the medicines (prescription, over-the-counter, and supplements) the child is taking.

When the laboratory reports the WBC count, it also reports the percentage of each different type of cell: neutrophils, lymphocytes, monocytes, basophils, and eosinophils. Normally, the neutrophils make up the greatest percentage. In young children (under the age of five), lymphocytes are often increased. Eosinophils are often increased in people with allergies. They may also be increased in children with parasitic infections. Certain uncommon rheumatic diseases (such as eosinophilic vasculitis, some cases of scleroderma, and Churg-Strauss syndrome) are also associated with a significantly increased number of eosinophils. Significantly increased numbers of monocytes or basophils are very rare.

Platelet count. Platelets are the sticky components of blood that initiate the formation of a blood clot when an injury to a blood vessel occurs. They are rapidly made in the bone marrow and the number may fluctuate quickly. The platelet count is often very high in people who are under stress or chronically ill. Kawasaki disease and iron-deficiency anemia are often associated with platelet counts over 600,000. Low platelet counts may result from certain medications. In addition, the platelet count may go down because of increased destruction in children with idiopathic thrombocytopenic purpura (ITP), systemic lupus erythematosus, Felty's syndrome, macrophage activation syndrome complicating systemic-onset JA, thrombotic thrombocytopenic purpura (TTP), or an infection. It may also be low because of decreased production in someone with leukemia, lymphoma, or aplastic anemia. At times there may be several different problems contributing to the low platelet count. If the platelet count is low without obvious explanation, the hematologist may recommend a bone marrow aspiration. This will allow examination of the cells that make platelets (megakaryocytes). If these cells are active, then the low level of platelets must be the result of increased destruction. If the megakaryocytes are inactive, there is decreased production of platelets. In addition, a bone marrow aspiration may provide clues to the cause of decreased production.

Erythrocyte Sedimentation Rate (ESR)

There are several variations of the ESR, but all of them reflect how the red cells (erythrocytes) interact with each other in the blood, as measured by how fast the red blood cells in a vial of blood settle to the bottom. During physiological stress (including but not limited to illness), the body produces proteins called acute phase reactants, which cause the red blood cells to move closer together and thus to settle to the bottom faster. Children with severe illness often have a high ESR, and this may prompt referral to a rheumatologist. However, in some people who are sick the ESR is not abnormal, and in some people with abnormal ESRs there is no obvious explanation. The normal ESR value varies with the age and sex of the patient and from laboratory to laboratory, so it is important to know the normal value for where your test was done. If the blood is left to sit for a long time or is not properly processed in the lab, the test is unreliable; this is why I look at trends and never act only on the basis of an isolated ESR value.

Whenever I am sent a child with an elevated sedimentation rate, I begin by taking a history and doing a physical exam to look for the reason the ESR is elevated. After that, I do further blood tests to look for other evidence of elevated acute phase reactant levels. It is important to investigate further until the explanation is found. However, in rare cases, children may have abnormal ESRs for which no explanation is apparent.

CRP

C-reactive protein (CRP) is an acute phase reactant that is made in the liver. Levels of CRP go up rapidly and come down rapidly, as well. Because the ESR (see previous section) measures a variety of acute phase reactants, the ESR and CRP generally move together, though the CRP may go up faster and come down sooner than the ESR. Many children who have rheumatic diseases, such as systemic-onset juvenile arthritis, have high CRP levels.

Chemistry Panel

The chemistry panel, also called the metabolic panel or serum multichannel automated chemistry (SMAC), consists of a variety of tests that document primarily the function of the liver and kidneys. In some hospitals, the test includes electrolytes and a lipid profile, but there is some variation between laboratories in the list of tests included.

Serum glucose refers to the amount of sugar in the blood. The level may be elevated or decreased in diabetics but is usually normal in children with orthopedic and rheumatic diseases. It may go up in children being treated with steroids. If the blood sample has been allowed to sit for too long before being processed, the value will go down.

Blood urea nitrogen (BUN) is a measure of kidney function. It is elevated in children with impaired kidney function. It often goes toward the top of normal to slightly over in children receiving nonsteroidal anti-inflammatory drugs (NSAIDs) because these drugs decrease the rate at which the kidneys cleanse the blood. These slight elevations are normal and should not be a cause of concern.

Creatinine (Cr) level is also a measure of kidney function, but it is not affected by mild changes in the GFR the way BUN is. Because children normally have lower creatinine levels than adults, the BUN/creatinine ratio may become elevated. This is not something to be concerned about if the underlying values are normal. One concern is that many laboratories do not report age-adjusted normal values. A creatinine of 1.2 mg/dl is normal for an older adult but very abnormal for a child under the age of ten. If the laboratory is not using age-adjusted normal values, the value of 1.2 mg/dl will not be indicated as abnormal in the child's results.

Sodium (Na), potassium (K), calcium (Ca), chloride (Cl), carbon dioxide (CO_2), and **phosphorous (P)** are electrolytes. Their levels may indicate abnormal kidney function or, under certain circumstances, other metabolic abnormalities. These should be normal in children with orthopedic and rheumatic conditions unless there is significant internal organ involvement. Like blood glucose and ESR, electrolyte levels are very sensitive to proper handling of the blood specimen and may be unreliable if the sample was mishandled.

Low sodium levels may be the result of fluid retention, brain injury, or medications. Children with very low sodium levels may have problems including weakness and muscle cramps, but values above 130 are rarely troublesome. High levels of sodium suggest dehydration or kidney disease.

Like the sodium level, the potassium level (K) is normally regulated by the kidneys. Low levels of potassium also cause weakness and muscle cramps. High levels may interfere with heart rhythm, and very high levels are dangerous. Low sodium levels with high potassium levels can occur in diabetics and in people who have poorly functioning adrenal glands.

Serum calcium measures the level of calcium in the blood. It may be abnormal in children with disease of the parathyroid gland, which secretes a hormone to regulate calcium levels. Sarcoidosis is a rheumatic disease that may cause elevated calcium levels. The level may also be abnormal in children with kidney disease, excessive vitamin D, or metabolic abnormalities. These problems may result in bone and joint abnormalities or pain if they persist for an extended period. Low calcium may be associated with severe muscle cramps. Rickets may cause problems in children who do not get enough vitamin D and is associated with a low serum calcium level and joint pains; however, rickets is extremely rare in the United States because most dairy products contain supplemental vitamin D.

Most often the serum chloride (Cl) level is normal. A very low chloride level can occur in someone who is sick and vomiting a lot. If you are dealing with a teenager who chronically has low chloride levels, you need to consider the possibility of bulimia (throwing up after eating to avoid gaining weight). Teenagers won't always admit to this unless confronted with the evidence. If an increased amylase level accompanies the low chloride, it strongly suggests the possibility of bulimia. The amylase comes from irritation of the salivary glands by the persistent vomiting.

Carbon dioxide levels in the blood go up and down as part of the mechanism that controls acid-base balance. If the CO_2 level is significantly off, a thorough metabolic workup should be done by the physician. However, the CO_2 level is another of the tests that may produce an abnormal reading if the blood specimen was allowed to sit for too long before it was processed.

Phosphorous is closely related to calcium metabolism. Children with kidney problems or calcium metabolism problems may have too high or too low a phosphorous level. Otherwise, the phosphorous level is rarely abnormal. Children who are using too much antacid may develop low phosphorous levels (hypophosphatemia). The antacids contain chemicals that bind the phosphorous in the intestines and prevent it from being absorbed.

Albumin is a serum protein manufactured by the liver that serves as both a building block and a carrier molecule. If the level is low, it may be the result either of decreased production from liver disease or poor nutritional intake or of increased loss through the gastrointestinal system or the kidney. In either case, it needs to be investigated. Systemic lupus erythematosus and amyloidosis are among many diseases that may cause increased loss of albumin through the kidney. This is easily detected by urine tests for protein.

Whenever the serum albumin level is low, the body must compensate by increasing other elements in the blood to maintain an appropriate osmotic balance. Most often the body increases the level of cholesterol in the blood to accomplish this. High cholesterol and low albumin are commonly found in children with kidney disease. Changes in diet are not likely to have any effect on these problems if the kidney or liver diseases that cause the problem are not corrected. If the body is not able to maintain an appropriate osmotic balance, water tends to leak out of the blood vessels, producing swelling. Painful swollen feet in children may be a sign of kidney malfunction and low albumin levels; sometimes the first clue is that socks are leaving deep marks on the feet or calves.

The chemistry panel also includes **total protein**, **total globulin**, and the **albumin-globulin ratio**. Globulins are larger proteins in the blood that include a number of acute phase reactants as well as immunoglobulin molecules. The level of acute phase reactants goes up in people who are ill, and so the globulin level goes up in people who are ill. At the same time, the albumin level often goes down when people are sick. The combination of factors often leads to a decreased albumin-globulin ratio. Low globulin levels also may be an indication of low immunoglobulin levels, associated with a variety of problems.

Bilirubin is commonly included in the chemistry panel. Most often it is reported as total bilirubin and direct bilirubin. The liver produces bilirubin from breakdown products in the blood. Direct bilirubin has been completely processed by the liver, while the total figure includes bilirubin that has not been so processed. Liver disease is the most common cause of significantly elevated bilirubin levels. If the bilirubin level is too high the child will look jaundiced, or yellow. In children with rheumatic or musculoskeletal disease, the most common cause of a significantly increased bilirubin level is hemolysis (the breakdown of red cells). This can occur after internal bleeding or if there is increased breakdown of red cells by antibodies. The latter complication, autoimmune hemolytic anemia, is often seen in children with SLE. Because red cells also contain an enzyme called AST (see next section), physicians may initially be confused into thinking that children with elevated bilirubin and AST levels have a problem with the liver, when in fact the liver is fine but too many red cells are being broken down.

SGOT/AST is an enzyme contained in muscle cells, liver cells, and red blood cells. Damage to any of these can result in increased amounts of AST being present in the blood. If the AST is elevated without obvious explanation, it is important to be sure that muscle enzyme testing (CK and aldolase) is done to look for muscle diseases, as well as a reticulocyte count to look for hemolytic anemia. Normal CBC and chemistry panels do not include the proper tests to look for these problems, and an elevated AST may be the only hint. But in a child with hemolysis due to excessive red cell destruction, the bilirubin level will also go up. This does not happen with muscle disease. If the elevated AST is the result of problems with the liver, there should be a significant elevation of the ALT as well (see next section).

SGPT/ALT is another enzyme that is primarily found in the liver. Thus, if the AST level is elevated but the ALT is not, it suggests that the source of the AST is outside the liver. Mild elevations of ALT can occur from disease outside the liver if the AST level is also elevated. There are many different liver diseases that may result in an elevation of the ALT level. The ALT level may also rise if the liver is being irritated by medications. Methotrexate is known to irritate the liver in some children, but NSAIDs and many other drugs may also cause liver irritation in some children. This is why it is important to monitor these tests routinely in children on medication.

It should always be remembered that some rheumatic diseases may cause damage to the liver, and some liver diseases may cause bone and joint discomfort. This is especially true in patients with infectious hepatitis. All children with significantly elevated liver enzyme levels need careful evaluation.

The level of **LDH**, lactic acid dehydrogenase, another enzyme measured in the blood, goes up with damage to many types of cells, including those in the brain, heart, lungs, liver, blood, muscle, or spleen. When there is increased cell turnover, the LDH level can be very high. Many physicians believe that an LDH level over 1,000 means that the child must have a tumor, but children with rheumatic diseases, such as systemic-onset JA or dermatomyositis, and other children with systemic illness may have very high LDH levels (well over 1,000 units). If a child is thought to have pauciarticular JA and the LDH is very high, something is wrong. These children should be evaluated for leukemia or bone tumors.

Alkaline phosphatase is an enzyme that is associated with bone growth. Because children have actively growing bones, the normal alkaline phosphatase value for children is much higher than the normal value for adults. If the laboratory is not reporting age-adjusted values, a normal value in a child may be reported as abnormal. In an adult, an elevated alkaline phosphatase may indicate gallbladder disease, but this is a rare problem in children. (Note that children with sickle cell disease can get gallbladder problems.) Occasionally, children have values of alkaline phosphatase many times the expected normal value without any apparent illness.

Uric acid is a breakdown product of DNA. Thus, increased uric acid means that either there is increased breakdown of cells or the kidneys are not properly clearing the uric acid, possibly both. Children sick with hemolytic uremic syndrome have high uric acid levels. So do children with leukemia. Sometimes children with elevated uric acid levels and joint pain are referred for possible gout. These children should be carefully evaluated for other problems. Gout is essentially unheard of in childhood except in the setting of kidney disease or cancer chemotherapy, where the drugs are causing many tumor cells to die very quickly and the kidneys cannot handle the load.

Muscle Enzymes: Creatine Kinase and Aldolase

Creatine kinase (CK) is an enzyme produced by skeletal muscles, the heart muscle, and the brain. Although it may be elevated in adults who have recently suffered a heart attack, the most frequent cause of elevations in childhood is muscle inflammation. This may occur in children with dermatomyositis, scleroderma, or mixed connective tissue disease. Sometimes the CK is elevated with extensive exercise, but in these children the level goes back to normal after two weeks' rest. The level of CK is also elevated after some viral infections. Some children have elevated CK levels that persist despite rest and for which no explanation can be found; see Chapter 14, on dermatomyositis.

Aldolase is another muscle enzyme that may be elevated in children with muscle damage. In general, the aldolase is less sensitive to muscle inflammation than the CK, but there are children with dermatomyositis who have elevated aldolase levels and a normal CK. Aldolase can also be increased in children with liver inflammation secondary to infectious mononucleosis or viral hepatitis.

Quantitative Immunoglobulins (IgG, IgA, IgM)

Immunoglobulins, the antibodies made to fight infections, are measured in the blood by the total protein but can be more precisely measured by specific tests. In a normal immune response, the body recognizes a foreign antigen and begins making antibodies against it by making IgM. As the immune response matures, the body begins to make IgG. IgA is also made in the secondary stage. There are additional antibody classes—IgE and IgD—that play a role in specific diseases.

IgG is the main class of immunoglobulin used by the body to fight infection. Without treatment, total deficiency results in death from infection. Partial IgG deficiency can take many forms, as there are several subclasses of IgG. If only one is missing, the child may have frequent infections, but otherwise do well. Children may also have a generalized low level of IgG; these children may have trouble handling viral infections and have an increased frequency of joint pains and limping episodes when they have viral infections. Defining these low levels is difficult, as large studies have shown that the normal levels of immunoglobulins in young children are highly variable. I have seen a number of young children (four to six years of age) with low normal levels who limp whenever they get viral infections. Thorough investigation has not found any additional abnormalities. As the children get older and their immune system matures, this stops happening.

IgA deficiency is an important special case of immunoglobulin deficiency. IgA is the body's defense against external bacteria at mucosal surfaces. Thus, IgA is found in the gut, in the saliva, and in the upper airways. Children with IgA deficiency have an increased incidence of colds and ear infections but in general do well. However, IgA deficiency is much more common in children with rheumatic disease than it would be if the two conditions were unrelated. It is important to recognize children with IgA deficiency not only because they have an increased incidence of infections and rheumatic diseases, but also because they can have major problems with transfusion reactions (see "Hypogammaglobulinemia-Associated Problems" in Chapter 7).

IgE is primarily associated with allergic reactions. High levels of IgE usually indicate a very allergic individual. They can also be found in children with eosinophilic vasculitis.

IgD levels are almost never measured. There is a very rare syndrome called hyper-IgD syndrome that causes children to have recurrent fevers and abdominal pain.

Specialized Tests

The **antinuclear antibody (ANA)** test determines whether serum from the child's blood reacts with various types of material in the nuclei of cells. ANA testing used to be very significant in diagnosing children with rheumatic disease.

The main problem with the test was that the results were difficult to compare between different laboratories. Each lab used its own materials for running the test and did its own calibrations. In the early 1980s it was decided that a standardized test would be better. A uniform cultured human cell line, called Hep2, was agreed on for the standard. But there are so many variables in performing ANA testing that it is still not safe to compare results between different laboratories. Furthermore, this cell line gives low-titer positive results (see below) much more frequently than the old method did. As a result, positive tests are now very common in children who do not have a rheumatic disease. Higher-titer positive tests are more meaningful. However, having only a low-titer ANA does not guarantee that your child does not have disease. As a result, the situation has become very confused.

Titer refers to how much the serum used in the test can be diluted and still give a positive reading. Serum is initially screened after being diluted at a ratio of 1:40. If the screen is positive, then further tests are done at dilution ratios of 1:80, 1:160, 1:320, and so on, until there is no detectable fluorescence. The last dilution at which the test is positive is the ANA titer.

Positive tests for ANA are found in a wide variety of conditions. They are certainly found in children with SLE, but they are also found in children with a wide variety of other rheumatic diseases including JA. They may briefly appear after a wide variety of infections (especially viral infections in which the virus has damaged the nuclei of the cells it infects). Positive tests for ANA have been seen in many children with no identifiable disease and in some children with many different diseases. The presence of a positive ANA should prompt consideration of a rheumatic disease, but it may be a false lead.

A positive test for ANA is also important in children with arthritis. In children with any of the various forms of juvenile arthritis, the complication of eye disease occurs more frequently in children who have a positive test for ANA than in children who have a negative test (see Chapters 5 and 6). Despite extensive investigation, the explanation for this association is unknown.

The pattern of ANA test results can be significant. Homogeneous pattern ANA occurs in many different people and is not disease-specific. Speckled pattern ANA is also common at low titer, but at higher titer it may be associated with mixed connective tissue disease or scleroderma. Rim pattern (also called shaggy pattern) is almost always a sign of active lupus.

The antibodies the patient's serum is reacting to during the ANA test can be extracted by a chemical solution. These antibodies are named Ro, La, Sm, and RNP. Different patterns of antibodies correlate with different patterns of disease (see Chapters 9 and 10).

Another early finding was that some of the antibodies detected by the ANA test were directed against DNA and that people with high titers of anti-DNA antibodies were often sicker. These tests used to be separated into tests for single-stranded DNA (ssDNA) and tests for double-stranded DNA (dsDNA). Tests for ssDNA have mostly disappeared, as these antibodies are very nonspecific and occur in a wide variety of situations. Most anti-DNA tests today measure dsDNA. High titers of anti-dsDNA are much more specific for lupus than a positive ANA. However, there are children with anti-dsDNA antibodies who have other diseases. Sometimes a child is very sick with a viral infection and anti-dsDNA antibodies appear as part of the immune response to the virus. These usually go away within a few months.

Many sources of DNA contain DNA in chains with damaged ends, which can cause positive anti-dsDNA test results that are not truly meaningful. A lab may run what's called a *Crithidia lucilliae* test, which uses as the source of the DNA a microorganism that has circular DNA, with no loose ends to be damaged. A positive test for anti-dsDNA antibodies using *Crithidia lucilliae* is more meaningful. However, even this test is occasionally positive in children who don't have SLE.

Antineutrophil cytoplasmic antibodies (ANCAs) are relatively newly described. Unlike antinuclear antibodies, which react with materials in the nucleus of the cell, these antibodies are reacting with elements in the cytoplasm of neutrophils (one type of white blood cell). The cytoplasm is the body of the cell surrounding the nucleus. There are two major variations: cANCA reacts with proteinase 3, and pANCA reacts with myeloperoxidase. With continued investigation it has become clear that pANCA may also represent antibodies to lactoferrin (a common protein) and other substances in the blood.

How and why pANCA and cANCA occur is unclear. Their importance lies in their association with Wegener's granulomatosis, pauci-immune glomerulonephritis, Churg-Strauss syndrome, other systemic vasculitis syndromes, and inflammatory bowel disease. If a child has unusual symptoms or symptoms that suggest one of these disease, the rheumatologist may test for ANCAs; if the antibodies are present, then more extensive testing is indicated. Unfortunately, the association of the antibodies with these diseases is incomplete. Some patients with the diseases do not have the antibodies, and some people with the antibodies do not have these diseases. As with so many other tests in rheumatic disease, we recognize the association but do not yet fully understand the how and why.

Anti–*Saccharomyces cerevisiae* antibodies (ASCA) are antibodies to a fungus that commonly occurs in the large intestine. These antibodies occur more often in children with IBD than in normal people. These antibodies are not routinely measured by rheumatologists but are increasingly being used by gastroenterologists in the evaluation of children who may have IBD. Studies have shown ASCA to be common in children with Crohn's disease, which is one type of IBD.

Serum complement levels. These tests are done in children with possible lupus. Although the complement system consists of many separate components, only C3 and C4 are routinely measured. C3 is typically depressed in children with active lupus and may be a warning of more active disease to come. However, the predictive value of a change in C3 level is the subject of much debate. There are few diseases other than lupus that cause a low C3. C4 is also frequently low in children with lupus. However, the significance of a low C4 is less clear. This is discussed in much more detail in Chapter 9. Many laboratories will also report CH50, but this is not a complement component. The test for CH50 measures the function of the entire complement system. If any one of the components of the system is low, then CH50 will be low.

C1q and C2 are two other complement components that can be measured, but these are not tested routinely. Genetic deficiency of C1q is associated with an increased risk of developing lupus. The risk of developing lupus is also increased in children who are deficient in C2 or C4. Deficiency of C4 does not cause any obvious illness, but deficiency of either C2 or C3 is associated with increased infections. Children with complete genetic deficiency of C3 often die of infections. Children genetically deficient in C2 have an increased incidence of infections and of rheumatic diseases but may live a normal life if they are recognized and given antibiotic prophylaxis. Most physicians think that C2 deficiency is extremely rare, but I have several children with C2 deficiency in my practice. You have to look for it to find it.

Anticentromere and anti-Scl-70 antibodies are associated with forms of scleroderma. Anticentromere antibodies are often present in children with CREST syndrome, and anti-Scl-70 antibodies may be present in children with systemic scleroderma. These antibodies are very significant if they are present. Most children who test positive for the antibodies will ultimately turn out to have the disease. However, I have seen false positive results and low-titer positive results that have turned out not to mean anything.

Like all diagnostic tests, tests for anticentromere and anti-Scl-70 antibodies are useful when they are done in children suspected of having the disease, but you must be very careful in interpreting them if they do not fit the clinical picture. Not every laboratory does these tests well. Before you get concerned about a positive test that does not make sense, make sure the test has been repeated in one of the nationally recognized laboratories (see the Resources section). Unfortunately, the absence of these antibodies does not guarantee that you do not have one of these diseases. They are found in less than half of affected patients and less often in children than in adults.

Anti-Jo-1 antibody is one of a variety of antibodies that have been described in adults with muscle disease. Some doctors still look for this antibody in children with muscle disease, but it is very uncommon in childhood. Adults with this antibody tend to have a more difficult disease course. There is a growing belief that patients who test positive for this antibody have a completely different disease from other patients with myositis.

Factor VIII, or Von Willebrand's factor, is one of the blood clotting factors. Someone who has no factor VIII has hemophilia (a serious bleeding disorder). In children with other types of inflammatory disease, the factor VIII level will rise and fall as an acute phase reactant. Some physicians like to follow this level in children with muscle disease or other diseases in which the blood vessels tend to be involved. A rising level suggests more disease activity, while a falling level suggests things are better.

Antigliadin antibodies, antitissue transglutaminase, and antiendomysial antibodies. Testing for these is done to detect children with celiac disease (gluten-sensitive enteropathy). This is an uncommon disease in which patients are sensitive to gluten, a protein in wheat and some other grains. Whenever they eat too much of this protein, they get abdominal pain and diarrhea. Interestingly, people with this disease develop arthritis and other autoimmune diseases more often than would be expected. Antigliadin antibodies can be of the IgG type or the IgA type. IgG-type antigliadin antibodies are very common and probably not meaningful. IgA-type antigliadin antibodies should raise suspicion of celiac disease. Antitissue transglutaminase and antiendomysial antibodies are much more specific indicators of celiac disease. Not everyone who tests positive has the disease, and a negative test does not guarantee the absence of the disease. However, these tests are helpful in deciding which children with abdominal complaints should be evaluated further. The definitive diagnosis of celiac disease depends on a biopsy of the small bowel that demonstrates the classic findings under the microscope.

Rheumatoid factor (RF). This test measures the presence of IgM antibodies directed against IgG in the blood. While the test is very useful in diagnosing adults with rheumatoid arthritis, the test is not often positive in children and should not be used to make the diagnosis of juvenile arthritis. RF is found in some normal people, people with a variety of rheumatic diseases, and in people with various infections, especially subacute bacterial endocarditis (SBE).

Adult-onset rheumatoid arthritis (RA) by definition occurs after sixteen years of age. However, since the disease does not always proceed as described in the literature, it occasionally starts earlier. So there are children with true adult-type RA that starts in the early teenage years, though this is not common. Children with certain infections, including SBE, also may have a positive RF test, as can children with other rheumatic diseases. A child with joint pain, a positive RF, and a positive ANA should be carefully evaluated for the possibility of scleroderma or mixed connective tissue disease.

You may hear about "hidden" rheumatoid factor. This is a very confusing subject. Typical RF is IgM directed against IgG. Because IgM has a unique structure that is very large, it is easy to detect these antibodies. Using special techniques, one can measure IgG and IgA antibodies against IgG, which are smaller and not detected by the normal RF test. These "hidden" rheumatoid factors are found in some children with juvenile arthritis. However, these tests are not commonly done, and their proper interpretation remains unclear.

Lyme titer. Lyme disease testing is a key element of the evaluation of any child with arthritis in areas where the disease is endemic. There are many different laboratories doing Lyme testing, and a variety of techniques are used. The easiest, least expensive test is the ELISA (enzyme linked immunosorbent assay), which identifies antibodies in the blood against spirochetal antigens. *Borrelia burgdorferi*, the agent that causes Lyme disease, is a spirochete; however, there are many spirochetes, some of which are normally found in saliva. If a child has Lyme disease, he or she will have a positive ELISA for antibodies to spirochetes, but so will many children who have been exposed to spirochetes other than

Lyme. All children with a positive ELISA should then be tested on a Western blot. The Western blot, a more complicated and more expensive test, determines exactly which spirochetal antigens the antibodies in the child's blood are reacting with. The Western blot can distinguish between antibodies found only in people with Lyme disease and antibodies found in people exposed to other spirochetes.

A child with a positive Western blot has definitely been exposed to *Borrelia burgdorferi* and needs to be treated for Lyme disease. However, that does not prove that Lyme is the cause of the child's symptoms, as Lyme disease and exposure to *Borrelia burgdorferi* are very common in many parts of the United States. If symptoms continue after treatment for Lyme, there may well be another problem.

Thyroid function tests are often done in children with joint problems because both excessive thyroid hormone (hyperthyroidism) and too little thyroid hormone (hypothyroidism) can be associated with diffuse aches and pains. Both hyperthyroidism and hypothyroidism also may be associated with fatigue and muscle weakness. In addition, autoimmune diseases such as SLE may be associated with antibodies that interfere with thyroid function.

The main thyroid function tests are T3 (triiodothyronine), T4 (thyroxine), and TSH (thyroid-stimulating hormone). T3 and T4 are hormones produced by the thyroid gland that regulate the body's metabolism. TSH is secreted by the pituitary gland and influences the function of the thyroid. In children with rheumatic disease, we occasionally see abnormalities of TSH without T3 or T4 abnormalities. This can be a warning of problems to come.

Some children with autoimmune diseases have high titers of antithyroid antibodies for a long period before they actually have thyroid disease. These may be antithyroid peroxidase antibodies or antithyroglobulin antibodies. Often children with antithyroid peroxidase antibodies have a family history of Hashimoto's thyroiditis. These children should be monitored carefully for the possibility that they too may ultimately develop Hashimoto's thyroiditis. Thyroid antibodies are also seen in some children with SLE and occasionally in children with celiac disease and other autoimmune diseases.

Serum protein electrophoresis (SPEP) is a test that measures the pattern of the proteins in the blood. A specific pattern indicates multiple myeloma, a cancer of the cells that make antibodies, but this virtually never occurs in children. However, the SPEP may detect IgA deficiency or a low level of other immunoglobulins.

Anticardiolipin and antiphospholipid antibodies were first noted in lupus patients with excessive bleeding, but it was discovered they were also present in lupus patients who had problems with excessive blood clotting (deep vein thrombosis, strokes, etc.). It turns out that these antibodies are present in some adults and children with a variety of rheumatic diseases as well as people who do not have any other identified autoimmune disease.

When these antibodies are found in someone who is not having problems with clotting, no one is sure what to do. It appears that most people with anticardiolipin antibodies are at very little risk, and it can be dangerous to give anticoagulants to people because they can bleed excessively if they fall, are cut, or are in an accident. Therefore, if the child has never had trouble with clotting, most doctors either do nothing or just give a baby aspirin daily. However, if a child has had a blood clot, most doctors believe he or she should be treated with anticoagulants.

Anticardiolipin or antiphospholipid antibodies can also affect pregnant women. Women known to have anticardiolipin antibodies should be carefully monitored when they become pregnant. Women who have an excessive number of spontaneous abortions (miscarriages) in mid- or late pregnancy often turn out to be anticardiolipin-antibody-positive.

PT and PTT. Routine clotting studies consist of two tests: the prothrombin time (PT) and the partial thromboplastin time (PTT). The PT measures the ability of blood to clot once it is exposed to thromboplastin (a substance that starts clotting). The PTT measures the ability of blood to clot when left out of the body without being exposed to anything extra to start clotting.

Anticardiolipin antibodies can prolong clotting, as can many drugs. Some children have prolonged clotting times because they either do not make or do not make enough of the clotting factors, which may be a genetic defect or the result of liver disease. Vitamin K is important for making the clotting factors, and someone who has prolonged bleeding should be given an injection of vitamin K. Surgery on children with an unexplained significantly prolonged bleeding time is dangerous.

HLA B27 is an inherited genetic marker. It is most common among people of northern European descent, but also is prevalent among those of Chinese descent and certain North American Indian backgrounds.

Eight percent of the white population is positive for HLA B27, and the vast majority of people are positive for this marker do not have arthritis. However, more than 90 percent of adults with ankylosing spondylitis have the marker. HLA B27 is also associated with Reiter's syndrome, the arthritis of IBD, psoriatic arthritis, and other forms of spondyloarthropathies.

Though we do not fully understand the operation of the gene that HLA B27 serves as an indicator for, we do know that HLA B27 signals a greater risk of developing arthritis given other circumstances. For example, if you have no other genetic predisposition to arthritis, being positive for HLA B27 is not significant. You may also have a genetic predisposition to arthritis that carries a certain likelihood that you will develop the disease. However, if you have the genetic predisposition plus the HLA B27 marker, your likelihood of developing arthritis doubles.

Urinalysis

Examination of a urine specimen (urinalysis) is the easiest way to determine whether the kidneys are inflamed or damaged. When damaged, the kidneys can leak red or white blood cells or protein. A typical urinalysis report will describe the **specific gravity**, which reflects how well the kidney is concentrating the urine. This must be evaluated with reference to whether someone has been drinking a lot or is dehydrated. If a person is dehydrated, the urine should be concentrated and have a high specific gravity. If he or she has too much fluid in the body, the urine should be dilute.

Sugar in the urine is called glycosuria. Normal people do not lose any sugar in the urine, but diabetics do. Children being treated with high doses of corticosteroids sometimes begin to lose sugar in their urine. If they do, it is an indication that they are moving toward diabetes and efforts should be made to reduce the corticosteroids. Another substance that may be found in the urine is **ketones**. Normally, there are no ketones in the urine. They are an indication that the body is metabolizing fat instead of carbohydrates. In someone who is sick or has not eaten well for a significant period, this is a normal finding. However, in a diabetic it may be a sign of significant trouble. Anyone with both ketones and glucose needs to be evaluated by a physician immediately.

Protein in the urine needs to be monitored carefully. Some people have orthostatic proteinuria, which means that their kidneys leak protein when they are standing for a prolonged period. This is a common and unimportant condition. This can be determined by checking a morning specimen. After lying down all night, they should not have protein in their urine. Other people have protein in their urine after a lot of physical activity, especially running. This is not significant either. However, people with nephrotic syndrome, a type of kidney damage, may constantly lose a lot of protein. This is determined by measuring the excretion of protein over a twenty-four-hour period or by comparing the ratio of protein to creatine in a urine specimen. Children with lupus may develop nephrotic syndrome. Children with amyloidosis, a rare complication of juvenile arthritis, often have protein in their urine and also may develop nephrotic syndrome.

Mild amounts of protein in the urine may be an indication that drugs or other chemicals are irritating the kidney. If protein appears in the urine after a new drug has been started, the situation needs careful monitoring. One problem is that certain NSAIDs are excreted in the urine and cause a false positive test for protein on a dipstick (quick) test. This can be determined by having the laboratory perform a more sophisticated test for protein in the urine.

Urobilinogen indicates the presence of bilirubin in the urine. This occurs only in the setting of liver damage or disease that results in an elevated bilirubin level in the blood. This may occur in children with hemolytic anemia because all the broken-down blood cells are metabolized into bilirubin. Another cause of a positive test for urobilinogen is the NSAID etodolac. When etodolac is excreted in the urine, it will react with the test strip and give a false positive test for urobilinogen.

Occult blood in the urine is hemoglobin from broken red blood cells. It suggests that there is bleeding somewhere in the urinary tract. This bleeding may be occurring in the kidney or further down the urinary tract. Most often this is associated with the presence of red blood cells. However, mild bleeding in which all of the cells are broken before leaving the body may show up only as occult blood. Another cause of a positive test for occult blood is **myoglobin**, a muscle breakdown product that is detected by the dipstick test for occult blood. Myoglobin can show up in the urine after muscle damage from crush injuries or even vigorous tackle football games. It may also be seen in newborn babies who had a difficult delivery. It is rarely present in children with dermatomyositis.

Small amounts of **red blood cells** in the urine may come from the kidney, the bladder, or anywhere else in the urinary tract. They may be present in the urine after vigorous exercise but should go away quickly. Investigation is necessary if a low level of cells is consistently present. Red blood cells can also appear in the urine if a child is struck hard in the stomach or on the back.

Some children with juvenile arthritis occasionally have blood in their urine without an obvious cause. Blood may also show up in the urine of girls during the time of menstruation. Sometimes a specimen is contaminated with blood just before a girl realizes her period has started. This is not a cause for concern. The specimen simply needs to be repeated after menstruation is over.

Most often a few **white blood cells** in the urine result from a specimen collected without proper cleansing beforehand. However, large numbers of white blood cells or clumps should be considered an indication of infection, and a urine culture should be performed. White blood cells in the urine may also result from irritation of the kidney.

Casts refer to clumps of red or white blood cells in the urine. They are called "casts" because the clumps take the shape of the urine tubules. If red or white blood cell casts are present, it is considered an indication of ongoing significant kidney damage. This is most often seen in SLE but can occur in other diseases that damage the kidneys. Hyaline casts are another type of cast but are not significant.

Bacteria in the urine suggest that either the specimen was not collected in a clean manner or that there is a urinary tract infection. If there is a urinary tract infection, it is usually due to a single type of bacteria, while a poorly collected specimen may contain many different types of bacteria. A leukocyte esterase test may help in detecting a urine infection, as the level of leukocyte esterase goes up when the white cells (leukocytes) are trying to fight an infection. However, this is not always a reliable finding.

Some compounds that are excreted into the urine by the body may condense into **crystals**. Uric acid crystals and calcium appetite crystals are very common. If there are a lot of these crystals, one must consider the possibility of kidney stones. These types of crystals are not normally associated with any of the rheumatic diseases.

Cerebrospinal Fluid Testing

Cerebrospinal fluid (CSF) is analyzed by performing a lumbar puncture, also known as a spinal tap. It is a relatively easy test in most circumstances. The only time it is unsafe to do a lumbar puncture is if there is increased pressure in the brain, which can be detected by examining the patient's eyes for evidence of increased pressure or by a CAT scan or MRI of the brain.

The fluid that is withdrawn from the lumbar puncture can be analyzed for evidence of infection, irritation of the brain, bleeding, or other disease.

In diseases such as lupus that may affect the brain, the child may start acting strangely. Often no one is sure whether the strange behavior is due to the drugs being used to treat the lupus, the child's being upset about being ill, the illness itself, or an infection. Examining the spinal fluid is the only way to be sure there is not an infection.

The report on the CSF will describe its color, which may be reddish or yellowish if there has been bleeding. If the tap is bloody, the doctors can tell by looking at the cells whether the blood is from the procedure or from bleeding in the brain.

In the absence of infection or irritation, there should be fewer than ten white cells per milliliter in the CSF. Large numbers suggest infection. Another check for infection is the gram stain. This is done by staining a drop of CSF on a slide and looking for bacteria under the microscope. Sometimes a child will have ten to twenty white cells per milliliter in the CSF. This can be from irritation or infection by a virus. It is less likely this is caused by a bacterial infection, but some of the CSF is always sent to the microbiology laboratory for culture just in case. In addition to the cell count the CSF is analyzed for the amount of sugar and protein present. The amount of sugar will decrease if there are bacteria in the specimen. A low sugar level and high protein suggest infection, but a high protein level with a normal sugar level suggests irritation.

Oligoclonal bands are another finding that suggests irritation of the central nervous system. They are sometimes found in lupus and sometimes in multiple sclerosis, but there may be other causes. If the doctors are worried about infections such as Lyme in the central nervous system, they will measure the concentration of antibodies to Lyme in the CSF and compare it with the concentration in the blood. Higher levels of antibodies in the CSF than in the blood suggest Lyme infection of the central nervous system.

23

Reconstructive Surgery

The goal of every pediatric rheumatologist is to maintain and restore the fullest possible level of function. In an ideal world, every child would receive proper medical attention early in the disease course and respond dramatically to therapy. Unfortunately, in the real world children do not always receive proper medical attention early in the course of their disease. In addition, some of those who do receive proper medical attention nonetheless fail to respond well. For those patients, our ability to replace severely damaged joints provides one of the most dramatic improvements in their long-term prognosis.

There are very few institutions that have the experienced surgeons and the necessary facilities to perform joint replacements on children and adolescents with rheumatic diseases. The Hospital for Special Surgery, where I work in New York City, has these specialized facilities, and children who need this surgery are often sent here.

At present we have useful replacements for hips, knees, and shoulders. We can also do useful reconstructive surgery on wrists, elbows, ankles, and feet. These surgeries often dramatically relieve pain and improve function. If a child's activities are being significantly limited by the damage to a joint, it should be replaced if possible.

ANESTHESIA

Whenever surgery is done, it is necessary to anesthetize the patient. Most joint replacement surgery used to be done under general anesthesia (the patient was put entirely to sleep and a machine would breathe for him or her). For children with severe arthritis, this was always a major problem. They frequently have neck involvement, and it is difficult (and sometimes dangerous) to put the necessary breathing tube in so that they can be put under general anesthesia. It was often necessary to do a tracheotomy (make an opening in the neck) so that the child could be properly ventilated.

At the Hospital for Special Surgery, today almost all joint replacement surgery can be done using regional anesthesia. This means that the child does not have to be ventilated by a machine. This eliminates the risks of injury to the neck that made it so complicated to do joint replacement surgery for children with severe arthritis in the past.

TOTAL HIP REPLACEMENT

Total hip replacement (THR) surgery is one of the most significant advances in the care of children with severe arthritis. Prior to the widespread availability of THR for children, any child with severe arthritis in the hip was simply placed in a wheelchair when the pain became too great. Few were ever able to resume walking. Now we are able to replace the hips of children with severe pain, and wheelchairs have become far less common.

Orthopedic surgeons with the experience necessary to do THR surgery on children are primarily found only in large academic centers with extensive experience in pediatric rheumatology. In addition, there are relatively few centers that have the sophisticated resources required to manufacture custom hip replacements for small children. The normal outcome of THR surgery is excellent. I care for a number of children and young adults who have had THR surgery. They could walk right past you on the street unnoticed.

The appropriate time for surgery is as soon as the child's arthritis begins significantly to limit his or her ability to walk around outside the house. If your child's hip pain is such that you are considering asking for a wheelchair, it is time to be asking for THR surgery instead. As soon as the child begins to use a wheelchair, he or she begins to lose strength in the legs and begins to develop flexion contractures in the knees. Both of these complications make it much more difficult to recover the ability to walk after surgery. The best outcome is obtained when the use of a wheelchair has been minimized or avoided completely.

Parents sometimes hesitate because they are concerned that the child will stop growing if the hip is replaced. It is important to remember that if the hip is so damaged and painful that the child cannot walk, proper growth is not going to occur anyway. Second, two-thirds of the growth in the length of the femur occurs at the end where the knee is. That growth is not affected by THR.

Other parents are concerned because they do not know how long the THR is going to last. It is true that the metal and plastic replacement assembly (prosthesis) may ultimately need to be replaced, but confinement to a wheelchair is not a better option. Hip replacements that become loose or otherwise need revision can be fixed repeatedly. The key is to have an experienced surgeon who is familiar with working with children. At centers such as the Hospital for Special Surgery, we have done surgery on children as young as nine years of age and as small as sixty pounds with excellent long-term results.

ARTHROSCOPIC KNEE SURGERY AND KNEE REPLACEMENT

Total knee replacement (TKR) surgery has been very successful in maintaining the ability of children to carry out their activities of daily living. With improved medications and the ability to suppress arthritis in the knees using intra-articular corticosteroids, TKR due to arthritis has become rare in children. Continuing active synovitis in a knee that has not responded to routine medications or intra-articular corticosteroid injection may be treated with an arthroscopic synovectomy (cleaning out the inflamed material through a small incision in the skin using a special instrument called an arthroscope). This therapy often provides significant relief but may have to be repeated.

Some children develop avascular necrosis in their knees as the result of corticosteroid usage. This is best treated with TKR. Usually, this does not need to be done in small children and does not result in significant loss of growth. As with hip replacements, knee replacements may need revision over time. However, experienced centers can do this when necessary.

ANKLE SURGERY

The ankle joint is difficult. The mechanics of the ankle joint are relatively complex and we have not found the mechanical replacements satisfactory. As of the time of this writing, it is generally better to fuse the ankle than to replace it. Fused ankles force children to walk without bending their ankles (it's clumsy, but it works). Because the joints of the ankle have been fused, the joints do not move, but they do not hurt, either.

FOOT SURGERY (TARSAL FUSION)

One of the more difficult problems for children with arthritis is involvement of the joints between the tarsal bones of the feet. These joints are important when you walk over an irregular surface or bend your feet. If they become significantly involved by arthritis, it may result in a lot of pain when walking. A surgical procedure called a triple arthrodesis will fuse these bones together. This results in a stiff foot and will cause difficulty when the child walks over an uneven surface, but it will relieve most of the pain.

WRIST SURGERY

The wrist is often significantly involved in children with psoriatic arthritis and some related spondyloarthropathies. It may also be involved in polyarticular-onset juvenile arthritis. There are two major problems. One is a wrist that hurts whenever it is bent. Some children get relief of their symptoms by wearing a splint on the wrist. If there is active arthritis, the splint may even result in the wrist fusing itself.

If the splint does not provide adequate relief, it may be necessary to fuse the wrist surgically. This is not a major surgery. The surgeon will fuse the wrist in a functional position to maintain its strength and functionality. If the wrist is not splinted or fused, there is a risk of progressive subluxation and deformity. When this happens, the wrist is permanently bent (usually downward) and loses function.

From time to time I will see children who are developing marked subluxation of their wrists. This causes the tendons that extend the fingers to rub on the end of the wrist bone on the little-finger side (the ulnar styloid). If this is allowed to continue, the tendons sometimes rupture and the patient loses the ability to open the fingers. An orthopedic surgeon can easily remove the end of this bone (the ulnar styloid), which should improve the situation.

SHOULDER SURGERY

The head of the humerus is called the glenoid. In some children with severe arthritis this can be damaged, limiting their ability to raise their arms over the head and perform other activities. This can interfere with dressing and other activities of daily living. Surgical replacement of the glenoid head is easily done in an advanced center.

24

Family Issues

Most of the parents reading this book will not have a child with a serious chronic condition. They can skip this section. However, if your child does have a significant disability, or you think your child's medical care is starting to take over your life, please read on.

If you have lived with a child with a chronic condition for any period of time, you know that this places a strain on everyone in the family. Any chronic childhood illness is not the child's problem; it is the family's problem. No one in the family is spared from the impact of the child's disease. Everyone will feel the impact of the attention diverted to take care of the ill child, everyone will feel the impact of the financial burden, everyone will feel the impact of missed vacations. Divorce and psychiatric disease are much more common in families of children with chronic illness than in the general population.

There is not going to be a single answer that works for every family. The one thing that is universally true is that ignoring the problem does not make it go away; it makes it worse. The successful families I see allow everyone in the family his or her own needs, the time and space to deal with them, and the ability to express feelings. This is what makes it possible for everyone to work together for the good of the whole family. Do not neglect your healthy children (or spouse) for the sake of the child who is ill. In the end, everyone will be unhealthy because of the psychological problems this causes. None of this advice means you should neglect the child who is ill, of course.

In many families, Mom is in charge of taking care of the children, including all the doctors' appointments and so forth. This can make her feel overburdened. The other children often start to feel neglected because of the time it takes for Mom to deal with the needs of the ill child. Dad often starts to feel neglected as well. This can cause big problems over the long term.

The families that cope most successfully do so by having everyone pitch in. Sometimes Dad brings the child to the appointment and Mom stays home with the other children. There will be times when everyone makes a sacrifice for the child with disease. Equally, there should be times when everyone gets to go somewhere special as a reward to make up for those sacrifices. Life is not fair, but it can be balanced. If you have several children, make sure each one gets the attention he or she needs. Don't forget to include yourself on the list of people who need attention and special activities.

It is not anyone's fault that your child has an illness. No one should feel he or she is being deprived or punished as a result. If you feel that your family is off to a bad start, sit down with everyone and talk about it.

Think about what you are going to do so that everyone feels attended to. You may need to call on your friends, relatives, and the local community. Do not be afraid to get help when you need it. There are psychologists, psychiatrists, and social workers who are trained specifically in dealing with the families of children who are chronically ill. I hope you do not need them, but if you do, ask your doctor. He or she knows how to get you help.

GROWING UP IS HARD TO DO

Another difficult situation for families of an older child with chronic disease is allowing the young adult to accept increasing responsibility and ultimately total responsibility for his or her care. Some hospitals have special adolescent clinics, while others sponsor specialized transition clinics for older children with chronic disease. But in most situations, if the physicians and family have done a good job of preparing them, as they get older the children will naturally make the transition.

When my patients obtain driver's licenses and begin to come alone to their appointments, they rapidly recognize their responsibility. Just as they can drive themselves to the appointments, they realize they are responsible for being sure that their blood tests are done in a timely fashion, the prescriptions are obtained or renewed, and their medications purchased. It's amazing how much more responsible they suddenly become when they can take themselves places.

There are physicians who feel that once patients reach a certain age, their care needs to be transferred to a rheumatologist or internist who specializes in adults. It is certainly true that patients need to be cared for by a physician who treats them in a manner that is appropriate for their age. If a physician is unable to adapt to their changing needs as they grow older, the patient should move on. However, many physicians are quite comfortable caring for patients of diverse ages. If the physician and patient have been working well together and trust each other, it is not necessarily in the patient's best interest to be forced to move on. I have learned a lot about how to deal with younger patients from my patients who have grown up and are now comfortable talking about how they used to feel. If you treat children as responsible participants in their own care from the beginning, nothing necessarily needs to change when they get older.

Some children with debilitating disease are forced to remain dependent on their parents even when they are clearly no longer children. This is always a difficult situation. Some continue to rely on their parents for all types of support, while others recognize that they qualify for appropriate aid for the disabled (such as Social Security disability) and assume responsibility for their own care. If the individual physician is uncomfortable providing the appropriate resources to deal with these issues, it may be best for the patient to be helped through the process by a multidisciplinary team in a transition clinic. Ask your doctor and local organizations what resources are available to you and pick the course that best meets the needs of your family. Do not be afraid to ask whether they have social workers available who can help you deal with the system. These people are there to help you.

DEPRESSION (PATIENT FATIGUE)

I have been discussing how hard it is to be the parent of a child with arthritis. What I have not talked about yet is how hard it is to be the child with arthritis or another chronic condition. When children are young, their problems are the responsibility of their parents. The children expect their parents to make them better. For most children with arthritis and related conditions, this is possible. The vast majority of the children I care for go on to live productive lives. However, the adolescent years of increasing self-awareness and increasing self-responsibility are difficult for everyone. They are even more difficult for children with chronic disease.

During the course of a chronic illness, there will be times when a child or young adult becomes depressed. He or she would be abnormal if this never happened. Parents and physicians need to be paying attention. While a certain amount of depression can happen to anyone, it is well known that some adolescents with chronic disease become suicidal. They feel that they have lost control over their lives and cannot see the light at the end of the tunnel. This may take the form of overt actions or simply failure to take their medications. Everyone should be listening for comments such as "It doesn't make any difference," "I don't care anymore," or "Why do I have to go to the doctor?" Parents and physicians must keep track of whether the medications are being refilled at appropriate intervals.

No one should try to tell adolescents with chronic disease that they shouldn't complain. It isn't helpful to tell them things could be worse. What adolescents need is someone with whom they can sit down and discuss their concerns honestly. It is important to acknowledge their problems while pointing out the positives and being proactive. If you are a parent and the doctor just gave you and your child depressing news in the office, talk about it. Don't leave your child to stew alone. Don't let your child hear you complaining about how hard his or her illness is for you, either. If you think your child is significantly depressed, ask for help. You might be depressed and need help, too.

There are psychologists and psychiatrists who specialize in dealing with adolescents and children with chronic illness and their families. Some children just need an honest conversation with their doctor. Others need an outsider to talk to. Some need medication. It is important to remember that there is no direct correlation between the doctor's opinion of how well or badly an adolescent is doing and the adolescent's opinion. Parents and physicians must be vigilant.

25

Getting the Best Results
for Your Child

This is the most important chapter of this book. Everyone wants the best results for his or her child, but not everyone understands that you have to go out and get them. Reading this book means you are off to a good start.

There are three major determinants of the outcome of any project: your level of effort and knowledge, the effort and knowledge of the people who work with you, and luck. No one can control luck, so it is very important to maximize your efforts and choose the best possible people to work with. First and foremost, you need a primary care physician you trust. If you simply picked your doctor from a book or you go to a group where you get a different doctor every time, make sure someone is listening to your concerns. If you think something is wrong with your child, make sure the doctor listens and examines your child carefully.

Few pediatricians have any training in muscle, bone, and joint diseases. Many think they have never seen a case of arthritis in childhood. Do not be afraid to press your concerns or to seek another opinion. Sometimes you have to insist. This book will help you determine whether there is really something wrong, but it is not a replacement for a good doctor.

CHOOSING A SPECIALIST

Once your primary care physician agrees that you need to see a specialist, ask him or her why you are being referred to the one chosen. You should be looking for the best doctor for your child. It may be the one in your plan, the one in the same building, the one in the same group, or the one in the same hospital—or it may not.

Ask the primary care physician whether he or she would take his or her child to the doctor who was recommended for your child's complaints. Ask the specialist about himself or herself. If the doctor is uncomfortable answering you or the answers make you uncomfortable, this might not be the right doctor for you. No one doctor is the right one for everyone.

Children with muscle, bone, joint, or arthritis pain often are sent to an orthopedist for a possible injury. If there is no history of an injury, be suspicious. Some orthopedists have little or no experience with childhood arthritis. I often see children with arthritis who were originally told they must have a hairline fracture that did not show up on the X-ray. If the problem promptly resolves itself, there is no cause for concern. However, if the problem keeps coming back, or there are repeated problems in many joints, a more detailed investigation is needed. This book will help you to know when you need to go further.

Finding a specialist on your own is not difficult. The Arthritis Foundation, the Lupus Foundation, and the American Academy of Pediatrics (see the Resources section) can direct you to the certified doctors in your area, but they may not be willing to recommend one over another. See which doctors are associated with the better hospitals in your area. In major cities, there are often newspapers or magazine articles reporting who are the top doctors. You can even find books listing the top doctors in America. While these lists don't always include the same doctors, those on these lists are likely well trained and well regarded in their specialty.

Unless you live in a very small town far away from any large academic center, you want a physician who fulfills the following criteria:

- Is board certified in the specialty
- Preferably is certified in the pediatric specialty (many specialists trained in internal medicine only rarely see children)
- Answers your questions in a way you can understand
- Takes time to explain what is happening
- Treats you and your child in a way that makes both of you comfortable

If the doctor recommended isn't in your insurance plan, you may want to consider whether it is at all possible for you to work with that physician regardless. Muscle, bone, and joint diseases are one area of medicine where the right or wrong decision now can make a difference for the rest of your child's life. In any case, find the best care you can.

AGGRESSIVE VERSUS CONSERVATIVE APPROACHES

There are "aggressive" and "conservative" physicians. What you want is a physician who is conservative when appropriate and aggressive when appropriate, not one who is always aggressive or always conservative. Some muscle, bone, and joint diseases tend to resolve over time. These are best treated conservatively. Some get steadily worse, and the longer you wait before you stop them, the more damage accumulates. You need a physician who can tell which is which and respond appropriately. The only way to know what your physician is thinking is to ask. Do not be afraid to ask questions.

SECOND OPINIONS

One of the most difficult issues for parents is when their child does not seem to be getting better. First, be sure you are doing what the doctor recommended. If you are, let the doctor know your concerns and discuss them with him or her. A good doctor knows that the child's health is the most important thing. If a family wants a second opinion, a good doctor will not act insulted. Instead, he or she will encourage the family. However, make sure you go to a well-qualified physician for the second opinion. Ask your doctor. If your doctor is confident, you will be sent to someone he or she believes is a valuable source of further information. If your physician is not confident, that may be all the more reason to go. Your relationship with your doctor is a major factor in determining your child's outcome. Make sure you have a good one.

CONFLICTING ADVICE

Parents feel immense pressure to make the right choice for their child. So what should you do when you get conflicting advice from two different doctors? Sometimes some of the advice is just plain wrong. However, far more often it reflects different points of view. Rheumatology is not a textbook science. If there were one correct answer, everyone in the field would agree and life would be simple.

As a physician, I can only make sure I explain the plan well, discuss the options, and explain why I prefer the option I recommend. In some situations, I recommend a course of treatment that is not in the standard textbooks. I see children from all over the world with difficult conditions who were sent to me because the answers in the textbooks didn't work for them. It is my job to offer the benefit of my experience and test new ideas. New therapies that work ultimately make it into the textbooks, but there are often delays of several years between when a new therapy is tested and found to work and when it is described in the textbooks.

Some physicians feel that it is up to the parents to decide which treatment plan to follow. They lay out all the options and say, "You choose." If physicians with all of their training cannot agree, how can the parents be expected to evaluate treatment choices? Physicians must not infringe upon the parents' right to choose for their child, but certainly doctors should accept the responsibility of recommending what they thinks is the best course. Parents, in turn, must decide what makes sense to them and which physician they are most comfortable working with.

There is no easy answer for parents who get conflicting advice. You need to know the doctors' backgrounds and level of training. Is one specialist widely respected in his or her field? Is the specialist someone who is teaching new physicians in the field? Ask these questions. If you ask enough doctors, sooner or later you'll probably find one who says what you want to hear. Is that the best therapy? Sometimes the advice that is most difficult to accept is what you really need to hear.

In the end, it is important to remember that you need to trust your doctor and have faith in his or her recommendations. If you do not, you need a different doctor. Unless you are working with a doctor who is not a specialist in the field, in most situations the quality of your working relationship with your doctor will have a greater impact on the outcome than most other factors.

FOLLOWING ADVICE AND KEEPING APPOINTMENTS

It may seem obvious, but following your doctor's advice and keeping your appointments are the most important things you can do for your child. All of us want to believe the problem will just go away if we ignore it, but when it comes to rheumatic disease and other chronic illnesses, ignoring the problem makes it worse.

All too often I see children who were supposed to be back in two weeks who come back in six months and still have the problem. Often the parents will say that the child took a few of the pills and then had a stomachache, so they stopped. Instead of calling the doctor to discuss the problem, they did nothing until everything got worse again. The more damage you let accumulate, the harder it is to fix. If you do not like the advice, call and discuss it with your doctor, or find another doctor. Prescriptions left in pockets or purses and pills sitting in bottles in the medicine cabinet will not fix the problem. You must take responsibility for getting your child proper care.

Every parent is concerned about the side effects of medication. This is a valid concern, because medicines do have possible side effects. But if the doctor thought the medicine was a greater risk than the disease, he or she would not recommend the medicine. You need to be sure that you are following up with your doctor and that he is monitoring your child appropriately (see Chapter 20). The reason for periodic monitoring visits and blood tests is to detect problems before they become obvious. Skipping your appointment because your child looks fine to you robs your child of the chance to have a problem detected before it becomes serious. Of course, most children don't experience side effects, but no one knows who will and who will not. By the time your child does not look fine, the problem may have progressed to a serious stage that is not easily reversed.

It's easy to skip the periodic monitoring appointments when your child is finally off medication. However, the same principle applies. We can never be sure a rheumatic disease is gone forever. If you did not notice your child's problems right away at the beginning, will you immediately notice them coming back? Your specialist is trained to detect the earliest signs of disease activity. Do you want to take advantage of his or her skills or rely on yours? The best results come when physicians and parents are both doing their part. You should take your child to all routine follow-up appointments. You should also bring your child to the doctor in between scheduled appointments if you suspect something is going wrong.

INSURANCE ISSUES

Dealing with insurance companies is one of the most frustrating aspects of medical care. They have no problem insisting that you make your premium payments each month. But somehow they often have problems paying you for your claims. Make sure your claim forms are properly completed and promptly sent in. Your insurance company will reject your claim for any mistake. Do not be afraid to call and ask where your money is. Good records are vital—keep a log of your phone calls, and write down the name and telephone extension of each person you talk to. Do not be afraid to ask for a supervisor. Do not take no for an answer.

Following up with insurance companies is a good example of the squeaky wheel getting the grease. Parents who keep after the insurance companies most often get paid. Parents who accept denials or small payments get what they accept. If you need a procedure or medication authorized by the insurance company, keep after them. I often have to get on the phone, and sometimes I have to speak to the medical director of the plan. However, you have to keep pushing the insurance company to move your appeal up the ladder. Your doctor cannot simply call them. They call the doctor when you've pushed them far enough.

Do not assume that the person on the other end of the phone has any real knowledge of your case. I've had medical directors of insurance companies tell me they did not know children could get arthritis. You are not dealing with a group of people who understand your needs and are concerned about your child's health. I've had representatives deny medications because they could not spell them. When I spelled it, the person on the phone said, "Oh, that's in my computer. It's okay."

When you are dealing with your insurance company, you are dealing with an organization that is trying to make a profit, which means reducing expenses. In many states, the appeal process brings in independent review panels. Often when insurance companies realize it is going to cost more to fight you than to give in, they will give in. You have to make them realize that you are going to fight for what you deserve.

DEALING WITH FRIENDS AND NEIGHBORS

To someone who does not have a child with a chronic problem, this section might sound unnecessary. However, all of us involved with children with serious diseases know how hard it is to deal with the questions and the stares when you are out in public with a child who looks or acts "different." Our number one goal as physicians is to make it so that no one will be able to tell your child has a problem, but we don't always succeed completely. The hardest part of this is that many people who stare or ask impolite questions are simply well-meaning and curious. As always, there is no easy way out. But this is one of those situations where practice makes perfect.

You shouldn't be worrying that you have to give your child's complete medical information to everyone who asks. In fact, you have no obligation to answer them at all. However, merely staring silently back in response to a question is likely to create an uncomfortable situation for everyone. I recommend that you make up an answer that is as short and simple as possible. When you are answering questions from strangers, it does not need to be true. I prefer simple, silly answers so that they realize you are politely telling them to bug off. Let's say a stranger asks, "Where did that red mark on your child's face come from?" You could answer, "That's where the Martians' rocket sled brushed against her as they were rushing to take off." Then turn around and go on with your business.

This same rule applies when your child is talking to adults and to other children. As your child gets old enough to talk to you about being asked questions, teach him or her what you have learned. First, make sure your child understands that the illness is not his or her fault. Make sure your child understands that the illness is not something "bad" about him or her. Then help your child practice a silly answer to give strangers. Encourage him or her to do this until your child is comfortable with it. Explain that the sillier the answer, the clearer it is that the problem is none of that person's business.

You do have to provide some information to your employer, your babysitter, your child's teachers, and other professionals with whom you interact—anyone who has some need to know. However, you still don't have to give the whole long story. I'm a strong believer in educating parents about the different types of arthritis and the different risk factors. But when you are talking to your employer, all you need to say is, "My child has arthritis."

The last thing to remember is that everyone needs someone to talk to. Don't brush off everyone in your life with the easy answers. It's up to you to decide whom you can truly confide in and take comfort from. If you find someone who is a good listener and supportive, you can confide whatever you think is important. You should explain this to your child as well. However, children are likely to get hurt because of this by someone at some point. It's a normal part of growing up. Try to help your child with deciding whom to talk to, and support him or her if problems arise.

DEALING WITH SCHOOLS

Many children with relatively minor disease escape having significant problems at school. But if your child has a chronic condition that is obvious to everyone, or even a mild condition that prevents full participation in physical education, the school will need to know.

There are a number of important things to know when dealing with your child's school. The most important is that the Americans with Disabilities Act put all the power on your side. If a few notes and an occasional phone call are all that is needed, it's great. However, if the school is being difficult, you may need an individualized education program (IEP), as described later in this section.

For most children with mild to moderate disease, everything can be handled easily. Often children need some leeway in physical education and perhaps a second set of books so they do not have to carry a heavy load of books back and forth to school. A quick note from the doctor's office is often sufficient. If there are going to be a lot of missed classes or if your child needs extra time to get from class to class or extra time on exams because of difficulty writing, you'll probably need an IEP. In most districts, this is not a major problem. However, IEPs take time and effort and often cost the school district money. The school administration may discourage you from asking for an IEP because it will "label" your child. If you are getting what you need, that's fine. Otherwise, push for the IEP.

If you need an IEP, the first step is a formal meeting at which you present your position regarding the needs of your child. You are entitled to have a parent advocate present with you at the meeting. Teachers, administrators, and counselors will also be there to help devise a good plan for your child. The school district is supposed to supply whatever is necessary to facilitate your child's education. Some parents go too far in making requests, but some school districts resist senselessly. You should certainly get your child's basic needs met. Do not be afraid of this process. It's designed with your child's best interests in mind. Moreover, the rules are slanted in your favor. But some school districts "forget" to tell you what you and your child are entitled to. Wise parents have spoken with their physician and other local resource organizations before the meeting. If necessary, there are even lawyers who specialize in representing parents at IEP meetings. Fortunately, they are rarely necessary.

SOURCES OF HELP

There are local and national organizations that can help parents of children with a wide variety of conditions. See the Resources for a listing. These organizations can be very helpful in directing you to other parents who have had similar experiences. They can provide useful information regarding the nature of your child's condition, experienced doctors, and other resources. They can also help you to find experts for dealing with the many problems of insurance, school, and so on. Many of the national help organizations now have Web sites as well.

THE ULTIMATE RESPONSIBILITY FOR YOUR CHILD'S OUTCOME RESTS WITH YOU

To provide the best possible care for your child, you must do some hard work. You must pick the right team, carefully choosing the doctors who take care of your child. Once you have chosen them, you must follow their advice. If you do not understand or do not like the advice, ask questions. Get answers. If you are not satisfied, get a second opinion. Then ask more questions.

Even after you have found a doctor with whom you are comfortable, you have not transferred the responsibility for your child's outcome to the doctor. You must make sure your child takes the medicine, does the exercises, keeps the appointments, gets the blood tests, and gets the treatments needed. It's not easy to find the time, to pay for it, or to take on the responsibility. But if you want the best outcome, it's not optional.

Appendix

There are thousands of organizations, Internet sites, books, and other resources for families of children with rheumatic diseases and related problems. There is no way I could list all of them here. I have listed the major organizations and others with which I have worked. I'm sure this list is incomplete. Many of these organizations have a Web page that may direct you to many others. My own Web page is http://www.goldscout.com. I regularly update the site with the latest information.

I have also listed some Internet-based groups that provide support for children with chronic illness and their parents. Be careful when you use the Internet: some of the information out there is excellent, but much of it is not reliable.

If you have time, energy, or resources left over after dealing with your child's problems, consider helping out with a volunteer organization. Some groups focus on improving research; others work on improving education about a particular condition, while others aim to improve access to care. Simply taking the time to talk to the parents of another child who has the same disease your child does can help when those parents are confused and uncertain where to turn.

ORGANIZATIONS DEDICATED TO HELPING CHILDREN WITH MUSCULOSKELETAL DISEASES

Organizations Without a Specific Disease Focus

National Institute of Arthritis and Musculoskeletal and Skin Diseases
Information Clearinghouse
National Institutes of Health
1 AMS Circle
Bethesda, MD 20892-3675
(301) 495-4484 or (877) 22-NIAMS (226-4267)
http://www.niams.nih.gov

U.S. Food and Drug Administration (FDA)
5600 Fishers Lane
Rockville, MD 20857
(888) INFO-FDA (463-6332)
http://www.fda.gov

American Academy of Pediatrics
141 Northwest Point Boulevard
Elk Grove Village, IL 60007-1098
(847) 434-4000
http://www.aap.org

American College of Rheumatology
1800 Century Place, Suite 250
Atlanta, GA 30345-4300
(404) 633-3777
http://www.rheumatology.org/index.asp

American Academy of Orthopedic Surgeons
6300 North River Road
Rosemont, IL 60018-4262
(847) 823-7186 or
(800) 346-AAOS
http://orthoinfo.aaos.org

Organizations Dedicated Primarily to Arthritic Conditions: Juvenile Rheumatoid Arthritis, Spondyloarthropathy, Ankylosing Spondylitis, Psoriatic Arthritis

Arthritis Foundation
P.O. Box 7669
Atlanta, GA 30357-0669
(800) 283-7800
http://www.arthritis.org
The American Juvenile Arthritis Organization (AJAO,
http://www.arthritis.org/events/ajao_programs_services.asp) is now part of the
Arthritis Foundation and may be accessed via its contact numbers.

Arthritis Society of Canada
393 University Avenue, Suite 1700
Toronto, Ontario M5G 1E6, Canada
(416) 979-7228
http://www.arthritis.ca

Arthritis Insight
http://www.arthritisinsight.com
This is a Web-based, question-and-answer site with information for children
and adults. The children's info is at http://jraworld.arthritisinsight.com.

Creaky Joints
http://www.creakyjoints.com
This is a site for children, teenagers, and young adults to share ideas, complaints,
and the knowledge that they aren't the only ones in the world with arthritis.

Spondylitis Association of America
P.O. Box 5872
Sherman Oaks, CA 91413(800) 777-8189
http://www.spondylitis.org
This group works with people with ankylosing spondylitis and with spondyloar-
thropathies.

National Psoriasis Foundation
6600 SW 92nd Ave., Suite 300
Portland, OR 97223-7195
(503) 244-7404 or (800) 723-9166
http://www.psoriasis.org

**Organizations Dedicated Primarily to Vasculitic Diseases: Systemic Lupus
Erythematosus, Scleroderma, Kawasaki Disease, Dermatomyositis**

Lupus Foundation of America, Inc.
2000 L Street, N.W., Suite 710
Washington, D.C. 20036
(202) 349-1155
http://www.lupus.org

Juvenile Scleroderma Network, Inc.
1204 West 13th Street
San Pedro, CA 90731
(310) 519-9511 (phone or fax)
24-hour help line: (866) 338-5892
http://www.jsdn.org

Scleroderma Foundation
300 Rosewood Drive, Suite 105
Danvers, MA 01923
(978) 463-5843 or (800) 722-HOPE (4673)
http://www.scleroderma.org

Raynaud's Association
94 Mercer Avenue
Hartsdale, NY 10530
(914) 946-5808 or (800) 280-8055
http://www.raynauds.org

Kawasaki Disease Foundation
9 Cape Ann Circle
Ipswich, MA 01938
(978) 356-2070
http://www.kdfoundation.org

American Behcet's Disease Association
PO Box 869
Smithtown, NY 11787-0869
(800)-7-BEHCETS
http://www.behcets.com

Sjögren's Syndrome Association
6707 Democracy Boulevard, Suite 325
Bethesda, MD 20817
(800) 475-6473
http://www.sjogrens.org

Myositis Association
1233 20th Street, N.W., Suite 402
Washington, DC 20036
(202) 887-0082
http://www.myositis.org

Organizations Dedicated to Other Diseases

Genzyme Corporation
500 Kendall Street
Cambridge, MA 02142
(617) 252-7500
http://www.genzyme.com/patient/patient_home.asp
Although this is a corporate Web site, it provides a wealth of information for patients with rare genetic syndromes that may be mistaken for rheumatic diseases: fibromyalgia, chronic fatigue syndrome, etc.

International Association for CFS/ME (Chronic Fatigue Syndrome and Myalgic Encephalomyelitis)
27 N. Wacker Drive, Suite 416
Chicago, IL 60606
(847) 258-7248
http://www.iacfs.net

Chronic Fatigue and Immune Dysfunction Syndrome Association of America
P.O. Box 220398
Charlotte, NC 28222-0398
(704) 365-2343
http://www.cfids.org

American Fibromyalgia Syndrome Association
PO Box 32698
Tucson, AZ 85751
(520) 733-1570
http://www.afsafund.org

National Fibromyalgia Association
2121 S. Towne Centre Place, Suite 300
Anaheim, CA 92806
(714) 921-0150
http://www.fmaware.org

Pediatric Network

http://www.pediatricnetwork.org

This site is intended for children with fibromyalgia, chronic fatigue syndrome, and related conditions and their families.

SPECIALIZED LABORATORIES FOR RHEUMATIC DISEASE TESTING

Rheumatology Diagnostics Laboratory

10755 Venice Boulevard

Los Angeles, CA 90034

(310) 253-5455 or (800) 338-1918

http://www.rdlinc.com

Specialty Laboratories

27027 Tourney Road

Valencia, CA 91355

(800) 421-7110 or (661) 799-6543

http://www.specialtylabs.com

Prometheus Laboratories, Inc.

9410 Carroll Park Drive

San Diego, CA 92121

(888) 423-5227

http://www.prometheuslabs.com

Mayo Medical Laboratories

http://www.mayomedicallaboratories.com

Multiple sites and phone numbers; see the Web page for details for your area.

MISCELLANEOUS RESOURCES

School-Related Resources

"A Guide to the Individualized Education Program by the Office of Special Education and Rehabilitation Services U.S. Department of Education," July 2000

http://www.ed.gov/parents/needs/speced/iepguide/index.html

Parent Advocacy Coalition for Educational Rights
8161 Normandale Boulevard
Minneapolis, MN 55437
(800) 537-2237 or (952) 838-9000
http://www.pacer.org

"Band-aides and Blackboards"
Joan Fleitas, Ed.D., R.N, Associate Professor of Nursing
Lehman College
Bronx, NY 10468
http://www.lehman.cuny.edu/faculty/jfleitas/bandaides
This site is dedicated to helping children with chronic disease and their parents
deal with school-related issues.

Information for Patients on Various Medical Procedures

Virtual Hospital
Total Hip Replacement: A Guide for Patients
http://www.uihealthcare.com/topics/medicaldepartments/orthopaedics/
hipreplace/index.html
Total Knee Replacement: A Guide for Patients
http://www.uihealthcare.com/topics/medicaldepartments/orthopaedics/kneere-
placement/index.html
Virtual Hospital has a variety of other useful pages found at http://www.vh.org.

Textbooks for Physicians

Anderson, Steven J., and J. Andy Sullivan, eds. *Care of the Young Athlete*.
    Rosemont, IL: American Academy of Pediatrics and American Academy of
    Orthopedic Surgeons, 2000.
Cassidy, J., and R. Petty. *Textbook of Pediatric Rheumatology*, 4th ed.
    Philadelphia: W. B. Saunders, 2001. This is the standard textbook. All of
    the rheumatic diseases discussed here are covered, with many references.
Greene, Walter B., M.D., ed. *Essentials of Musculoskeletal Care*, 2nd ed.
    Rosemont, IL: American Academy of Pediatrics and American Academy of
    Orthopedic Surgeons, 2001.
Isenberg, David A., Patricia Woo, and P. J. Maddison, eds. *Oxford Textbook of
    Rheumatology*, 2nd ed. Oxford Medical Publications. New York: Oxford
    University Press, 1998.

Other Books for Parents

Aldape, Virginia Tortorica, and Lillian S. Kossacoff. *Nicole's Story: A Book About a Girl with Juvenile Rheumatoid Arthritis.* Minneapolis, MN: Lerner Publications, 1996.

Horstman, Judith, William J. Arnold, Brian Berman, J. Roger Hollister, and Matthew H. Liang, eds. *The Arthritis Foundation's Guide to Alternative Therapies.* Atlanta: Arthritis Foundation and Longstreet Press, 1999.

Lane, Nancy E., ed. *The Osteoporosis Book.* New York: Oxford University Press, 1998.

Lockshin, Michael. *Guarded Prognosis: A Doctor and His Patients Talk About Chronic Disease and How to Cope with It.* New York: Hill & Wang, 1998.

Wallace, Daniel J. *The Lupus Book: A Guide for Patients and Their Families.* New York: Oxford University Press, 2000.

Wallace, Daniel J., and Janice Brock Wallace. *All About Fibromyalgia.* New York: Oxford University Press, 2002.

Index